Slices of Life

After Traumatic Brain Injury

Slices of Life after Traumatic Brain Injury
©2015 by David A. Grant.

Produced in the United States of America. No part of this book may be used or reproduced in any manner without written permission whatsoever except in the case of reprints in the context of reviews.

This book does not dispense medical advice. Brain injury is a serious medical condition requiring treatment by medical professionals.

For more information, write to:

Professional Media Services, PO Box 236, Salem NH 03079

On the Web: www.DavidsNewLife.com

All Rights Reserved.

To my Wife Sarah

And my Loving Parents

Table of Contents

Learning to Crawl

9. The Slow Crawl of Brain Injury Recovery
13. Unusual Brain Injury Symptoms Abound
16. Living with TBI & PTSD
24. A Whale of a Good Time!
28. Reeducating a Damaged Brain
33. The Day I Met Little Bear
41. Get a Group, Get a Life!
47. Why Mince Words? PTSD Sucks
53. Life: Predictably Unpredictable
57. Getting Back on the Bike
61. The Journey Continues
65. I am Disabled

Learning to Walk

70. Hi God, it's me, David
73. Developing Compensatory Strategies that Work
79. An Unexpected TBI Teaching Moment
84. Traveling at the Speed of Light
88. Reclaiming Intimacy

94. Learning to Live in the Moment
98. Developing a Meaningful Life
106. No Two Paths are Alike
108. The TBI Zone
113. Watching Out for Rogue Waves
117. TBI Injustices
121. Let's Talk about Fear
126. Dead Man Walking

Learning to Soar

131. To Infinity & Beyond!
136. A Brain Injury Milestone
141. I Have a Secret
145. Developing Effective Adaptive Strategies
149. Living an Unfiltered Life
153. Where There's Life, There's Hope
157. To Share or Not to Share
163. Of Fireflies and Thankyous
168. Building a Life after Brain Injury - Let's Get Social
173. From a TBI Meltdown Comes New Hope
177. Building a Survivor Family
182. Metamorphosis
187. Post Traumatic Growth

Introduction

In 2010 my life changed forever. The teenage driver who struck me while I was cycling in my home town was barely old enough to shave. Bones were broken, flesh was torn and I entered the strange and surrealistic new world of traumatic brain injury.

I started chronicling my journey as a brain injury survivor very early on with my first written piece completed a short 48 hours after my accident. Little did I realize that I was laying the foundation for my first book, *Metamorphosis, Surviving Brain Injury*.

The years continued to pass and I did what I do best, I wrote – often in painful and heartbreaking detail about my life's struggles as a brain injury survivor. But time passed and my journey became easier. Never easy, but easier.

Looking back, I realized that I had an immense body of written work that offered a feel for what life is like as a true survivor. Each written piece is strong in its own right, but woven together as a collection, readers will come away with an insider's perspective about what life is really like for brain injury survivors and those who love them.

There are three distinct segments in this volume, *Learning to Crawl, Learning to Walk, and Learning to Soar*.

In *Learning to Crawl*, readers feel the pain of early life after traumatic brain injury redefines life. *Learning to Walk* demonstrates that the first few steps can be hard, but can indeed be mastered. In *Learning to Soar,* the magnificent reality that a meaningful life can be lived after a brain injury is revealed.

Recovery from a traumatic brain injury cannot be measured in days, weeks or even months. Recovery is lifelong. No longer do I look at recovery as "getting back" to the life I once had. Rather, recovery to me is now defined as coexisting with my brain injury. I have slowly learned that there will be good days – days that I cherish, and there will be hard days – that will always pass.

It is my hope that you will find hope in this volume of essays, that you may better understand the degree to which a brain injury affects not only the survivor, but all who know them. And that you will come away with a new belief that, though forever changed, a meaningful and fulfilling life after TBI is possible.

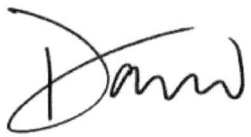

Learning to Crawl

The Slow Crawl of Brain Injury Recovery

"The beginning is the most important part of the work."
~Plato

So much of life happens between those moments of normalcy. The sun rises, the sun sets, many of us go to work, care for our children, spend time with those we cherish and never give much thought to the fact that life can change dramatically in the blink of an eye.

And so it was in November of 2010. For it was on a cold, blustery late-fall day in New England that my life was forever changed. Local police estimate the speed of the teenage driver who broadsided me while I was cycling at 30-40 MPH.

In two ticks of a clock, my life unexpectedly and abruptly changed course. I was thrown from my trusty bike into the strange new world of traumatic brain injury.

Never did I know the scope of how large traumatic brain injury is in today's society. Called by many, *America's Silent Epidemic*, I was blissfully unaware that over 3.4 million Americans a year sustain a traumatic brain injury.

Recovery from a brain injury is like nothing I have ever experienced. If you are a survivor, you already know this. I you are a family member or a caregiver, you know this as well. But to live life as a brain injury survivor, there are no past experiences I can draw upon that have helped me as I navigate through this new and uncharted life territory.

In the days after my cycling accident, I saw doctors of all shape and form. The orthopedic doctor let me know that my broken arm would heal, that I would be casted for a couple of months and feel a bit of pain for six months. Right on cue, at the six month mark, my arm pain stopped.

But recovery from a brain injury cannot be defined by an end-date circled hopefully on a calendar, though I thought this at first. As my broken body began its slow crawl toward wellness, as my bones knitted, and as my bruises faded from black to yellow and then to memories, the extent of how my brain injury was affecting my life began to become clearer.

My journey to my "new normal" may or may not be typical. Brain injuries are like snowflakes- no two are alike. In the days after my injury, I had a CAT scan, an EEG as well as other tests to see if my cognitive abilities were compromised. I passed all my early tests with High Honors and was congratulated by many within the professional community for dodging a bullet.

But all was not well. Most all of my symptoms, those cues that let me know I had sustained a TBI, came slowly, in many cases weeks after my injury. Word-finding issues were among my first challenges. Then came significant challenges with my memory. We can add to the list a couple of new-found speech impediments: stuttering and aphasia.

Yes, on the outside, I "looked" normal. But under the hood, it was becoming very clear that something was wrong.

Another trip to the neurologist revealed a new, multi-facetted diagnosis. Grateful that my body was mending, and still confused over some of my newest challenges, I was told I have a very clear-cut case of Post-Concussive Syndrome. Adding more to the list, it was at this same time, by now several months after my accident, that I was also diagnosed with Post traumatic Stress Disorder.

My nature, how I am hard-wired, is to be a problem solver. I am an overcomer. Whenever a life event comes to pass, the optimist in me tries to pull whatever positive I can from the experience and move one.

But with a brain injury, there is no end-game. There is no magical date on some future calendar page that is circled in red, perhaps with a smiley face, that I await. I have learned over the last couple of years that recovery from brain injury is lifelong. I have learned that the brain recovers in its own time, sometimes at glacial speed. And if I try to hurry the process, I am left disheartened and frustrated.

Life as a brain injury survivor is vastly different than I ever expected. Challenges I never gave thought to in my old life can overwhelm me. Akin to learning to drive a new car, I am slowly learning how to navigate through life with my new limitations.

But there is good news.

By being respectful of my new limitations, and surrounding myself with people who love me, who care about me and who want me as well as I can be, a new life can be built after a traumatic brain injury. Yes, much of it is more difficult. But much of it is surprisingly more wondrous. I have slowed down to a pace I never had before and now take time to see, feel and experience my world with deeper appreciation than I ever thought possible.

And for that, I am profoundly grateful.

Unusual Brain Injury Symptoms Abound

"It's easier to resist at the beginning than at the end."
       ~Leonardo da Vinci

Many of the events that have come to pass since my accident are simply surrealistic.

Take, for example, my new inability to feel cold. Since Impact, my ability to feel cold has all but disappeared. Never having been overly fond of winters here in New England, at first glance, this may sound like a quite a blessing.

Like many of my long-term symptoms, the awareness that something changed, that something internal shifted, came slowly over time. There was no ah-ha moment, just a gradual realization that something was different; that my new normal had just shifted again.

It was a sunny day in March of 2011. Like I have for many years in March when the weather cooperates, I decided to wash my car in the driveway. A bucket full of suds in front of me and a garden hose by my side, I looked the part of most any weekender partaking in giving my car its ritualistic bath.

Basking with the sun on my face, my body slowly healing from the accident 5 months prior, I noticed longer than normal stares from folks driving by our home. Living on a busy corner, rubberneckers come with this territory. Folks watching what kind of flowers we plant, eyes glancing over as the lawn is being cut, it's all part of life on a corner lot.

But there was something different that day. Very different.

The stares were just a little longer. Cars passing by at a fraction of their normal speed. Like I had done hundreds of times before, I was washing my car in shorts and a t-shirt. No shoes on my feet, my footsteps marked by soap suds in my driveway. This was not, however, a typical car-washing spring kind of day. You see, it was sunny day, but it was not a warm day. The thermometer topped out at only 38 degrees, though I knew it not.

My ability to feel cold had shifted. Sometimes there is no sensation at all when it's cold. Sometimes I feel cold like pain. There is no sensation of any temperature change. Rather, my arms, legs, hands and feet hurt in response to cold.

Odder still, sometimes I feel cold as the color white. This is difficult for me to describe as it defies traditional logic.

One thing for sure about this new life, it certainly is unpredictable.

Living with TBI & PTSD

"Even when we have hardships, we can be very happy."
~Dalai Lama

I watched her sleep today. Always the first one up in the morning, my brain often waking up an hour or more before I do, today I had the luxury of not jumping tight out of bed.

And she was smiling in her sleep.

And I was glad... glad that she was able to find a measure of peace away from the daily challenges of life.

We've all heard that old saying about a picture being worth a thousand words. But looks can indeed be quite deceiving. A face smiling back at you as you look at a picture tells you so little. Rather than a using picture to tell the tale, today I opt for the Thousand Words.

A little over two years ago, on a day too much like today, the old David died. Thrust through time and space in an obscene montage of glass, metal and bike parts, I soared through the air and into the new and often unfathomable world of traumatic brain injury.

I feel the need, at some level beyond my ability to describe, to chronicle my journey. Like an unscratched itch, if too many days go by without pen to virtual paper, I just get nudgy.

Why write? The reasons are myriad. I write to create a tangible record of my journey, one that I hope to look back on with delight as I see forward progress. As many of my new friends are in the same TBI club I am in, I open my heart and soul in an effort to let others know that they are not alone... that others share in their challenges and truly understand.

And I write so that I can try to better understand my own new life, to capture a perspective I can gain no other way. My goal today is to offer a bit of a snapshot as to what my day-to-day life is like as I start year three of life since my accident.

A brain injury is like a shadow on a sunny summer day. It follows you everywhere you go. No matter how fast you run, no matter how high you jump, there is no escaping your shadow. My TBI dogs me much the same way. It's always there. Sure, there are moments that I don't think about it. Like that summer shadow, you know it's there. Just look down and you'll always see it. But it never goes away.

Ever.

Ask most anyone with a TBI what words are the most likely to raise the hair on the back of their neck and they will more often than not say something like, "but you look normal." Brain injury is often called a hidden disability. Most who may see a picture of me and Sarah would be inclined to thing we look like a couple of fun people out living life. To a large extent, that's true, but there is so much more.

These days, my challenges, while very familiar, still abound...

Of the day-to-day challenges that have become part of the ebb and flow of life, it is the Post Traumatic Stress Disorder that continues to be the most challenging. Two, three, or more nights a week I wake up either screaming, shaking, or with a face covered in tears, my body wracked with uncontrolled sobs. This past week alone, my mind after dark has seen me in the company of one of my closest friends as he prepared for his own suicide. He lost his wife, his soul mate, his best friend three years ago. I was close to him while she faded away to cancer, and have been a steadfast friend since she passed into the Realm Beyond. In yet another PTSD night terror, he let me know it was time to join her. The pure vividness of my PTSD nightmares simply cannot be described. He looked into my eyes and said goodbye, thanked me for being there for him, for being a true friend. I watched the tears stream down his face as he knew he was both saying goodbye and getting ready to see his beloved wife again. I wept with him.

And awoke in the instant before he died.

If there is any silver lining to this one, it was that I woke up without waking up Sarah. A while back she said that life today was like life with a newborn in the house. How well I remember those days, walking around mind numb from 2:00 AM feedings. Doing your best with a head clouded with a sleep-debt induced fog, to focus on the awake part of your life, only to know that there was another night coming with questionable, if any, sleep. Such has been the nature of our lives for over two years. And it tears at my heartstrings, knowing that my issues effect Sarah. Don't let anyone kid you. Brain injury effects virtually everyone involved. Wives, husbands, mothers, fathers, children, the list goes on. All are impacted by a TBI.

Always one to live in the solution, I have tried everything the "professionals" have suggested and more. A year of therapy did not eliminate the PTSD nightmares. A well-intentioned doctor offered prescription medication that almost took my life in the form of my own suicide, so medication is off the list. When the neuro-psychologist said no caffeine after 2:00 PM, I was obedient almost to a fault. We can add to this list little or no technology at night. How about chamomile tea as was suggested? I still drink chamomile tea every night... and we've seen how well that works. As only the desperate can relate with, I did have a healing session with a Native American healer at a Pow Wow this past summer. And for two blessed weeks, I slept. Week three brought about the same-old-same old. A dream catcher now hangs over my bed. Last night was the second night in a row of blessed sleep. And it's bittersweet. I cherish the sleep but know that every night of no nightmares means I am closer to my next bad night. Those who know me know that I am positive by nature, so this is more of simple stating a truism, than anything. It is what it is.

Other challenges abound. I can no longer tolerate crowds for any length of time, and situations that are unfamiliar can fill me with an anxiety heretofore unknown to me. The list goes on... from unending tinnitus to my inability to perceive the passage of time, life is often surreal, often hard and often painful. Last year, Sarah gave me a watch with a very clear month, day, and time presentation on the watch face. Even still, I look many times daily at my watch to see whether it's March or November, only to forget where I am in the timeline of life and look again... and again.

Lost is most of my ability to remember where I stand in the realm of time. It's one of those odd quirks of a head trauma that is difficult to even begin to explain. If you see me somewhere, and I do nothing more than smile and say hello, perhaps banter about the weather a bit, you would never know what life is like behind the smile. But I do. It's one of those frustrations I try not to even think about, as nothing can be done about it.

But all is not a veil of tears.

Though all of this, I have been introduced to some of the most inspirational people I have ever met. People whose lots in life make mine look like a cake-walk. Other TBI survivors are on the short list of some of my closest friends. I have met caring professionals who are truly compassionate in their care. I've had complete strangers reach out to me with kindness after reading my book. The list goes on.

And I have changed. It's hard to wrap words around some of the changes, but I'll do my best.

Philosophical feels like the best word today. More than before my injury, I am inclined to look at the extremes. The Bigger Picture is now clearer to me. At times, I can rise above the din of daily life, look around and "see" with my soul's eyes in a way I never knew possible. And the smaller things in life have taken on new meaning. I find myself wrapping my arms around Sarah several times a day. Not needing any type of reassurance, I find simple pleasure in just holding her. A sunset can now stop me dead in my tracks. My near-death has slowed my pace, and often that is good thing.

My life is changing. My internal compass has spun around a few times and is beginning to point in a new direction. And I am setting new goals; some very personal to me, and others in the realm of where I want to go in the next chapter of my life.

Time has already shown that my experience as a TBI survivor makes me uniquely qualified to help other TBI survivors. I "get it" from an insider's perspective and have had real-world experience in rebuilding a post-TBI life. While it makes me feel naked by putting so much of myself out there, it helps other souls. I feel a deep sense of moral responsibility to use the voice that I have.

And I am pushing forward developing a new career as a writer. Prior to my accident, my written work had seen national publication on several occasions. But my voice has changed and has evolved... and is stronger and more compassionate than it was in my pre-accident life.

It's been 743 days since my life changed forever. And in those 743 days, over 3.5 million American's have suffered a head injury. That is million with an "M." The numbers are simply staggering.

Like I have done countless times over the years, today I baked brownies. Sarah and I have an errand to run. The brownies as well as a couple of signed copies of my book are heading over to our local Fire Station. Our town's first responders are part of the reason I am still here. And I shine a light of gratitude on them in my book for their service to our community.

While they may not remember in the same degree of clarity that day a couple of years ago that they scraped up an injured cyclist off Main Street, it is a day I will never forget. And today, brownies, still hot, will cross the threshold of the fire station.

And again, I will say thank you.

A Whale of a Good Time!

*"Only when we are no longer afraid do
We begin to live."*
~Dorothy Thompson

If you have a brain injury, or know someone who has, you know firsthand that life can be difficult at best. And downright impossible on those "bad TBI" days.

Call me odd, but there are a few things about my TBI that are actually fun. It's taken me years to get to the point of even being able to say this.

I look at it this way: My life changed forever when I was struck while cycling back in 2010. I can either make the most of what I have or spend non-recoverable time lamenting the death of my old self.

For so many of us, our collective TBI experience marked a sudden and unexpected death of who we were. But so often, from death springs forth new life.

Be mindful that I said a *"new"* life. Not an *"easy"* life. Or even a *"familiar"* life.

We get what we get and time marches on.

At a year after my TBI rebirth, I found myself going through extensive neuropsychological testing. Not ordered by an insurance company or even a lawyer. No, this was a fact-finding mission for Sarah and me.

Simply put, it was time to see how many cards I had left in the deck. If I was going to be short a couple of Aces, so be it. Best to know my deck was a bit light than be surprised at the end of this poker game called life.

I'll spare you more of the doctor's visit details. You can read about that in my book if you so choose. (www.metamorphosisbook.com)

This gifted doctor said I had lost my problem solving ability. He went on to say that I was permanently disabled and that I had tested out at the bottom of the testing barrel for problem solving.

This actually explained a lot. Things that were familiar to me before my TBI were often still within reach. Not always easy, but doable. But I had known for quite a while that new things, new events, new life challenges... well, they left me profoundly confused.

While some folks may have made the decision at this point to simply *"stick with the familiar,"* Sarah and I opted for a dramatically different spin on this. If new things were going to come hard, then bring it on. We've all heard that old adage, *no pain, no gain.*

Earlier this year, my wife Sarah & I sat down and wrote out a month-by-month list of something new we would do every month. Amazingly, we are working through the list. And BOTH of our lives are enriched because of this.

On our new to-do list in July of this year was to be a Whale Watch off the New Hampshire coast. Having vertigo as part of my new life, the mere thought of being on a boat gave me more than a bit of anxiety. As the recipient of four new letters in my life- PTSD, I need to always have an exit strategy from just about anywhere. How exactly does one exit a small boat thirty miles offshore?

Last July found us face-to-face with a 60' fin back whale. As this amazing creature spouted water skyward, Sarah and I found ourselves bathed in what I now fondly call whale snot.

And it was amazing on so many levels.

Fear was walked through. I told my PTSD to take the back seat for a little while. And we had the chance to see something few others see, whales frolicking in the Wild.

Still, you might be wondering what I meant when I said there were things I actually liked about my TBI. (Or, if you are like me, you might have already forgotten already that I even said that...)

When the ship's captain said it would take an hour and a half to get to where the whales would be found, more than a couple of my fellow travelers rolled their eyes.

But since my brain injury, time as I knew it went away. I have lost most of my ability to effectively discern the passage of time. While most had to wait out the time, in my new TBI world, an hour and a half feels like only 10 minutes.

I smiled and waited for my own personal 10 minutes to pass, and enjoyed my new whale of a friend.

After an hour or so watching this magnificent creature, we started the trek back to the New Hampshire shore.

It was an easy ride back. It only took 10 minutes!

Reeducating a Damaged Brain

"An investment in knowledge pays the best interest."
~Benjamin Franklin

No one really likes to think about brain damage.

Sure, around these parts, we talk a lot in initials. TBI, ABI, MTBI, EEG, PTSD, MRI... the list goes on.

But the reality in my world is that when I sustained a traumatic brain injury, I experienced brain damage. There is no way to candy coat this harsh reality of what happened. I was struck while cycling, broke bones, torn tendon and ligaments, bruises in places I never knew possible, and I sustained brain damage.

My dis-inhibition these days means that I am far more likely to be more candid than ever. I try hard to always temper my comments and to never indict harm or pain.

There is an immense freedom in this soul-level honesty.

Fourteen months ago, a leading neurologist was part of my continuing education about TBI. While I have read many books, browsed volumous of web-content, and become a bit of a sponge as I learn about TBI, most of my real-life knowledge about life with a traumatic brain injury comes from living it. If you have a TBI, you know exactly what I mean.

This same neurologist shared a fact that didn't sit well at the time. In fact, it scared me witless.

"Your IQ has dropped since your accident. It is very common among brain injury survivors to see a degradation in intelligence."

At 14 months post-impact, I was still in fact-finding mode. Still trying to figure things out. Trying to make sense of something so overwhelmingly surreal that it felt like a bad dream. One that I was unable to wake up from.

And thus this trusted doctor became yet another actor in the screenplay of my life.

Like most new news that hits me hard, I took it in, held my head high at his office... and cried all the way home.

Degradation of intelligence?

As this fact settled in, my first reaction was purely self-pity. Oh, how I would love to say I embraced this news and carried on. But that was not the case. I stewed about it for a while.

And somewhere, from deep within, the fighter began to emerge.

Before my accident, I had a long history of beating things. It was clear that I was not going to be a victim of his diagnosis.

I remain as committed to cycling and wellness today as I was before I was hit. Daily I cycle thirty or more miles. Most every day. I am one of the lucky ones. While I crash mentally most days at 2:00 PM, I can still rife.

But I made a decision. Rather than listening to two hours of music on my MP3 player, it was time to try something new.

I shared with Sarah that I was going back to school for a Liberal Arts degree... and that I was going to pay no tuition.

From that day on, my two hours a day on my bike with my ear buds in became a bit different. While I occasionally choose music on the weekends, my new Monday through Friday audio track is now vastly different.

My daily playlist now includes regular current events podcasts from NPR. I have listened to hundreds of hours of American Academy of Sciences "Science

Podcasts." Simply put, we become what we are exposed to. I am pumping new information into my brain at a speed unlike anything I have encounter since college.

So how is this informal education working?

As my memory is not what it used to be (a vast understatement) some of what I hear is quickly forgotten.

But much of it sticks. In fact, I am often shocked at how much I do remember. I've developed a bit of a fascination for astrophysics. Of course, anything related to neurology captures my interest in a heartbeat. I've listened to hours of Grammar Girl podcasts that have helped me with my writing. The list goes on.

The take-away is this: I was made aware of a new deficiency that resulted from my brain injury. Rather than simply accept that "it is what it is," I opted to try something new.

And it paid off.

I don't want to leave you with the impression that I don't have "stuff." Living with a TBI is the hardest thing I have walked through- ever. It is unending, uncomfortable, terrifying, unpredictable... the list goes on.

But this is my only life. And I am doing the best I can to deal with this. And a few hundred hours of podcasts later, I can tell you about amazing things like exoplanets.

I will continue to push myself hard. Harder that I probably should.

But I owe it to myself and those close to me to get as well as I can.

The old David is gone and the new David is still a bit unknown to me.

But so far, he seems alright.

The Day I Met Little Bear

*"Humankind has not woven the web of life.
We are but one thread within it."*
~Chief Seattle

It was the last place I ever expected to be. I had reached the point of pure and unadulterated desperation. Half way through year two as a traumatic brain injury survivor, life as I knew it was more painful than anything I had ever experienced. I had reached the jumping off point. Thoughts of suicide were rampant and I was quickly running out of options.

He introduced himself as "Little Bear" as he handed me his business card. The title on his card?

Native American Healer.

In an effort to maintain some semblance of normalcy, Sarah and I did our best during those abysmally tough first two of years after my brain injury. We continued to do many of the things we did before I was hurt.

One of our favorites remains unchanged to this day. So often, we'll hop in my car and drive north to the White Mountains of New Hampshire. There is something healing, something cathartic about being at one with nature. Away from the daily hustle and bustle of life, away from traffic and shopping malls, our trips to the North Country always leave us both re-centered.

So it was only natural that the North Country would call to us during this difficult time.

Passing a roadside sign almost too small to see, the words *Pow Wow Today* caught my eye. A quick u-turn found us pulling into the parking lot – with events unimagined about to unfold.

For a reason I still can't explain to this day, I left my shoes in the car, and chose to walk through that fated day barefoot and connected to the Earth. Some of the best things in life happen when you are barefooted. Sarah and I were married in bare feet, but that is a tale for another time.

A small kiosk at the entry to the tribal grounds collected a voluntary donation. There was an air of spirituality that was palpable. From the smell of burning sage that hung heavy in the air to the sound of drumming off in the distance that seemed to resonate through the Earth itself and run right up my legs to the core of my broken being, something holy was in the air.

I watched people approach the kiosk. As a brain injury survivor, I am invisibly disabled. But those approaching the kiosk wore their disabilities with honor. I watched young parents pushing a child in a wheelchair. People hobbled in on crutches. A couple of Downs' kids were among those I first saw. The list goes on. Like pilgrims to the Ganges River in India, they came to be healed.

And in two ticks of a clock, I knew at the level of my soul that I was supposed to be there that fated day.

At a year-and-a-half into my new life, I was in the toughest shape of my entire life. So many brain injury survivors who had been walking this new path longer than me let me know the same thing – the first couple of years were going to be the hardest. They also shared that it would get easier. I just never imagined it would be so hard.

So, what kind of shape did I find myself in at the eighteen month mark?

My dual diagnosis was that of a TBI as well as Post Traumatic Stress Disorder. At eighteen months, my PTSD was kicking my backside. The wail of an ambulance siren more often than not would reduce me to uncontrolled tears. But far worse than that were the nightmares. Three to four nights a week, I would awaken whimpering, screaming or crying hysterically from nightmares of all makes and models. My wife Sarah did her best to coax me back into the land of the living and away from the daemons in my head. She would fall asleep and I would lay there in abject terror wondering what was coming next. I wrote in exquisite detail about this time in my recovery in my book *Metamorphosis, Surviving Brain Injury*. Truth-be-told, it's tough for me to look back and read about it to this day.

Daily I would walk around in a perpetual state of sleep debt and nightly, I would come to great harm in my sleep. Almost from the get-go, I had made the decision that I would go to any lengths to get as well as I could, to do all that I could to live successfully as a brain injury survivor. I never had expectations about getting back to my pre-brain injury self, but I was determined to get as close as I could.

Slowly I learned that I could sometimes simply coexist with my brain injury, while at other times, we get into the ring together, put on the boxing gloves and spar for a round or two.

From cognitive therapy to a great support group; from a well-intentioned psychologist, to devouring everything I could read, nothing seemed to work for my nightly trips to Hell and back.

Such was my condition on the day of the Pow Wow.

A Native elder was smudging those wishing to be healed. I stood in line, eyes filled with tears. How did I get here, to this point of sheer desperation?

Sarah and I spent the next couple of hours walking the grounds, watching the Grand Procession, breathing in all the positive energy and enjoying the healthy distraction from the living torture life had become.

Heading back to our car, we passed a tent with sign outside.

Native American Healer, read his sign. His prices for sessions were listed below.

Five dollars for fifteen minutes.

I stood there for a few minutes, Sarah by my side. Like me, she was weary. Like me, she was trying to understand her new role as the wife of a brain injury survivor.

"Do you want to try this?" she asked with just a hint of encouragement. She knew my state. My state was "our" state.

Sheepishly and a little embarrassed, I said yes. Heck, what did I have to lose? Five bucks is not a bank-breaker.

The tent flap opened and out came a man ten years or so my senior. He looked gentle. He looked kind.

I can't tell you all that happened inside his tent. Not that I don't want to, I simply don't remember it all. We talked for a couple of minutes. He asked me what I was looking to be healed from.

And the water-works started. I told him about my brain injury. I shared that nothing worked. I told him of the nightmares, of dying in my dreams – in ways I won't detail here. My dreams were as traumatic as my brain injury.

He shared that he had been in Viet Nam and had seen unspeakable events. And he shared that he was now whole.

Eyes closed as this twenty-first century medicine man performed his ritual, a ritual most likely that has been passed down through the ages, I could feel the bass beat of the drummers through my core. Soft words were chanted in an unfamiliar tongue and incense burned.

Eyes wide as I emerged from his tent, I flipped him a ten.

"I don't need change." I thanked him and went off to find Sarah.

By now you are most likely wondering if this foray into the realm of the non-traditional had any affect.

For the next two weeks, the nightmares completely disappeared. I slept as I had not slept since my brain injury. I would love to share that that was the end-game for my PTSD nightmares, but it was not. A couple of weeks later, they came back with a vengeance – and remained with me for the next year.

Gratefully, at two-and-a-half years after my brain injury, my nightmares abruptly dissipated. A medical professional called them *"self-resolving."* These days, now well into year four since my TBI, I might have one or two bad nights a month. Comparing this to where I came from, I am quite OK with it.

Like so much that encompasses living with a brain injury, recovery timelines are measured not in days or even weeks, but in years.

Just the other day, Sarah and I passed the tribal grounds where these events came to pass. The gates were closed and two feet of snow barred any entry.

I couldn't help but smile at the memory of that day in July of 2012.

I am grateful to no longer live in Nightmare Alley. And I am grateful that I have experienced full-blown PTSD. That may sound odd, but my experience means that I can better understand others who fight similar battles.

And that alone means that my challenges were not in vain.

Get a Group, Get a Life!

"A real friend is one who walks in when the rest of the world walks out."
~Walter Winchell

While still in my first year of life after my brain injury, I was told about a newly forming support group for brain injury survivors at a nearby rehab hospital. The first meeting was to be held in April of 2011. And I was a perfect candidate for the group.

In over the half-century that my life has spanned thus far, I've seen amazing wonders. I've seen all four of my own sons take their first breath.

Nothing can hold a candle to watching lava flow down Kilauea at night and roll into the sea in billows of steam. From sunsets over the desert to simply watching my wife Sarah as she sleeps, I have experienced joys unimagined.

But like any other human being since the dawn of time, hardship has reared its head repeatedly. From the unexpected loss of family members to a bankrupt business, some heavy blows have fallen. This does not make me unique. It simply makes me human. I carry no hard feelings or resentment about any of my challenges or difficult experiences. In fact, at a deeper level, I can appreciate them as they strengthen me. As steel is tempered and made stronger by fire, so have the fires of my own life, including my brain injury, made me stronger.

And long ago I learned an important life lesson. Problems carried alone are problems doubled while problems shared are problems cut in half. Looking back over the most difficult challenges in my life, those times that I was part of a peer group of others with similar experiences were dramatically easier than those times I tried to go it alone.

Such was my life experience and mindset when I learned of the new TBI Support Group.

I am blessed in that the rehab hospital is only a short ride from our home. In fact, the ride over is under five minutes. Arriving for the first meeting ten minutes early, I found an easy parking space, grabbed my notebook and started a new part of my journey I am walking to this day.

A bit of a perspective check is in order. Until that first meeting, I have never knowingly met someone with a brain injury. My understanding of my injury was just beginning, and my awareness of my newfound limitations was growing. Virtually all of my knowledge up to this point in time was presented to me by well-intentioned doctors, by books I had read, and by information I had found online.

I can recall that first meeting like it was yesterday. Walking into the conference room, I was both anxious and excited. Having no idea what to expect, I was a proverbial blank slate when I arrived. And life was about to again change.

A couple of folks sat at a conference table. After poking my face through the door, and seeing what appeared to be just a couple of staffers engaged in conversation, I mumbled something about having the wrong room. As I started to exist stage left, one of the attendees called to me.

"If you are looking for the brain injury group, you've found it."

Truthfully, I'm not sure what I was expecting. Wheelchairs? People with visible challenges? I was completely both out of, and in my element at the same time. I can look back on it now and smile as I "look" normal. Just as my newfound friends did.

Over the next few minutes, the room slowly filled with people. People who look just like you, just like me. It's not called America's Silent Epidemic without just cause. By the time the meeting started, there were a dozen of us there, brought together by a shared tragedy, and now bound together by an unasked for life experience.

The facilitator took a couple of minutes to explain a bit about the group, talked about the direction the group may go in, and started the dialogue by asking each of us to share what had happened. And the stories that unfolded that night were breathtaking. Stunning events had come to pass for everyone there that night.

One by one, we shared what happened.

From the young college student who had hit a tree while skiing to tale after tale of auto accidents, I sat there spellbound. There was even a cyclist like me who was injured by an errant driver. So much for being unique.

Yes, the causes of the injuries were as different as wildflowers in a meadow. But what shocked me were the tales of life after tragedy. Here were a group of people who shared challenges I had never before heard articulated by another soul. From speech problems to memories that no longer functioned, from incessant tinnitus to chronic exhaustion, I was among those who knew of these things not from reading about them in books, but from actually living life with a brain injury.

Initially scheduled for an hour, our first meeting went over by about ten minutes. Simply put, no one wanted to leave. There was an immediate sense of comfort, a palpable sense of peace that came from simply being in the presence of souls with similar fates.

Though I only had a five minute ride home after the meeting, I made the decision to take a long-cut and not head straight home. My head was spinning. I was no longer alone in my challenges. That night I met people who have long since become my friends.

And I cried.

The water works started before my key even found my car ignition. I cried like I had never cried before. The pent up fear, frustrations, anxiety, apartness and more all came out. Red rimmed eyes met Sarah at the door that night. She looked at me, said not a word, and embraced me.

We meet once a month at the hospital. There have even been get-togethers at some of the homes of the regular members. And I've never missed a meeting.

I cannot overstate how critical, how cathartic and how vital to my own recovery this meeting has been. And it's grown. We have newer members who drive (or are driven) from 20 - 30 miles away to be part of this cherished group. Though I have quite intentionally tried to forego giving any direct advice, I am going to deviate a bit here. If you are a brain injury survivor, please find a group. You'll thank me for it.

Over the last year, we've had guest speakers, hours and hours of face-to-face sharing and a new Facebook Group has started letting us stay in touch between the monthly meetings.

And yes, there is a perennial box of tissues at our meeting, often making its way up and down the full length of the table at every meeting.

Why Mince Words? PTSD Sucks

"PTSD is a whole-body tragedy, an integral human event of enormous proportions with massive repercussions."
~Susan Pease Banitt

Hanging on the back of our bedroom door is a calendar.

Just like the kind you see everywhere, there is a section under the date to add a note, mark a birthday, or simply write a little reminder. At first glance, it all looks pretty average.

But like the very fabric of life, looks can be deceiving, so very deceiving.

Looking closer you'll see one of two notations on every date. Every date is assigned one of two cryptic notes. You'll see either a smiley face or you'll see the letters N.M. Turn back the pages in time over this past year, walking backwards through the year through November, October, September and hop, skipping and jumping all the way back to January, you'll be hard pressed to see a day without one of these two notes. We can travel back in time through the now dusty 2011 calendar and see the same notations- ad infinitum.

You may be wondering the significance of this.

Sarah, my best friend, lover, hand-holder, sharer of half my heart, constant companion as we walk though this life... Sarah has taken on an unasked for role as she chronicles my PTSD. The smiley faces mean that the night prior was a good night. That I fell into restful sleep, my arm wrapped around her until morning. This is the way life is supposed to be. She wakes up, heads over to the calendar and dully notes a good night with a smiley face.

So what does N.M. mean?

Grab on to your seat and hold on. Time for a peek behind the curtain. Follow me to the dark side.

Three months after my accident, I was diagnosed with PTSD. So much of our post-accident life is defined by letters. MTBI, PCS, ABI, PTSD.

Just like there are a myriad of flavors of ice cream, so it is with Post traumatic Stress Disorder. No two cases are alike. Unlike so many, I can bike by the exact spot where my soul was bruised in a cacophony of broken glass, twisted metal and wailing rescue vehicles... I can pass that exact spot, and do several times a week, without any real issue. Sure, there are still times I bike up Granite Ave and think to myself, *"This is where I experienced the last few minutes of a life I now mostly forget."*

So many others are haunted my ghosts of memories of the actual event that caused their own PTSD.

But my personal nightmare manifests mostly after dark. When the world is getting ready to slumber. When boys and girls are getting ready to visit the Land of Nod. That is when my own personal daemons start their warm-up rituals and wait for me to fall asleep.

The N.M. on the calendar, so deftly annotated by Sarah refers to those nights I wake up screaming in terror. Afraid for my life. Covered more often than not in sweat and sometimes unable to stop shaking. Over the last year, each month has seen between ten and fifteen notations of N.M. on our ever-present calendar

N.M.

Night Mare.

And yes, today's date on the calendar is not marked by a smiley face.

1:30 AM this morning. *"Wake up, David..... wake up.... please wake up,"* her arm over me, trying to pull me back into the realm of the living. Into a world where it is safe. And away from my night terrors. Some nights I pull out of it quickly. Eyes wide open, panting, but present. Then there are nights like last night. My dreams won't release their stronghold and coming back is difficult. My terror wrapped around me like a noose, trying to strangle all hope from me.

The common theme, the corrosive thread though most of my night terrors involves my imminent death. Most are so richly textured and vivid that they feel over-real. But the worst ones, the ones that all but guarantee that I wake up in tears, involve harm to Sarah. Words cannot describe what it is like to wake up in the midst of such overwhelming anguish or grief.

"Still I find this narcolepsy slide...into another nightmare." ~Third Eye Blind

The timeline is stunning. I am now well into year three since my life was shattered. And there has been no measurable relief.

Those who know me know that I am a chronic over-comer. I beat things. Not much is beholden of the power to hold me back for long. Not even a brain injury. But I need to share that this one is kicking my butt.

Always and ever the obedient patient, I have heeded all medical advice. This time last year, I was just winding down on a years' worth of therapy, to no avail. Also suggested and tried: no caffeine after 2:00PM, limited or no technology in the bedroom, chamomile tea, hot showers before bed, winding down my day with a period of mediation. Hitting my knees bedside begging the Power behind the Universe for a measure of relief for the upcoming night.

Yet, again last night, like the night before... and many other nights just this month alone, my nightmares torment me.

I have made the decision again to reach out into the professional community to get help. I have met many doctors along this new road- some good and some abysmal. My neuropsychologist has a recommendation for a new PTSD specialist. I will be in touch with him next week.

How I wish that was the end of this chapter, but there is so much more...

As our health insurance is strictly a catastrophic plan, with a deductible high enough to buy a decent car, the first step is to see if the new doctor is "in the budget." As my accident has left me working only part time, life is different. Smaller. Funds are tight and tough decisions have to be made. I rarely experience envy. Blessed beyond measure, Sarah and I have each other. There is food in the fridge, and she is in the kitchen baking holiday cookies as I write this. But man o' man, what I would give to have traditional insurance, to pay a co-pay, see a good doc, and not worry if it became a choice of the mortgage or health care. Just this month, I made the final payment toward the medical debt from my accident 2+ years ago. It felt like I had paid off a small mortgage.

Sarah has offered to dip into her retirement fund to pay for any needed healthcare. I have adamantly said no. Yes, we have today, we also have to care for our future. And will for the rest of our lives.

Why share in such vivid detail? There is an easy answer. Brain trauma is not an episodic occurrence. There is no, *"get it, treat it and move on,"* reality to all this. This is a chronic condition that even years later requires care. And I know from many of the new friends I have met along my new road that the challenges I face are faced by countless others. Called *America's Silent Epidemic* with 1.7 million new TBIs in the US annually, I willingly put a face on this. I raise my voice so that others can learn.

Sarah and I will do what we have done since the get-go. We'll talk, hold hands... prop each other up and continue to move forward.

Life: Predictably Unpredictable

"At its best, life is completely unpredictable."
~Christopher Walken

Getting used to living with a traumatic brain injury takes time - lots of time. Years ago I heard shared what so many of us have heard, *"Recovery from a brain injury is a lifelong experience."* I have to admit, that really didn't bother me that much. When you really dig deep, most of us are recovering from something.

But the real eye-opener was how long it has taken me to realize that the light at the end of the tunnel is not a train. I am beginning to experience moments of life being okay. It has taken years.

While there isn't a lot that's really comfortable about living with a traumatic brain injury, there is an element of predictability to it all. I've been dancing this new dance with my brain injury for long enough to know how it feels. My dance partner, perennially paired with me on the dance floor of life, is predictable.

I can expect to live daily with brain fog. That's part of our new TBI two-step. I can expect to have bouts of overwhelming exhaustion. Occasional vertigo and speech challenges are part of this new life as well.

Word finding after a long day can be like playing hide and seek with my vocabulary. Now you see it, now you don't.

The point I'm trying to make is that for quite a while, years in fact, this is the only existence I know. Where living with a damaged brain used to be unnatural, it's now my normal state. Somewhere that Winnie-the-Pooh voice that narrates the timeline of my life just said to me, "David continued to grow, sometimes quickly, sometimes slowly, as he wandered the Hundred Acre Wood of his mind."

Early on, had you or anyone shared that this degree of acceptance would slowly permeate my being, you would have been met with a resounding "never." Recovery is a process, not an event. And most every day, I proceed a bit deeper into my new life.

But there is a bit of an unexpected pendulum effect to all this. One that swings from the realm of the predicable, through its arc, into the realm of the unpredictable. Shared before and most likely to be shared again, there are two links in the chain that defines so much of my new life as a brain injury survivor.

The first link is my brain injury. The second link is another newfound friend - Post Traumatic Stress Disorder. They are forever bound together, forged as one by the hammer and anvil of my cycling accident back in 2010.

As predicate as my brain injury is, my PTSD is equally as unpredictable. It keeps me on my toes.

My wife Sarah and I live in Southern New Hampshire. Our town has three Fire Stations with one being only a few blocks from our home. I can hear the wail of sirens a few times daily as our first responders heed the call of duty. There are many times that an ambulance can wail by our home and I don't even give it a second thought. In fact, I barely even notice.

But at times unexpected and unpredictable, that same sound can reduce me to tears, leaving me paralyzed, unable to move, with eyes full to the brim with tears. There is no rhyme or reason. Now you cry, now you don't. It is predictably unpredictable.

My old friends, Mr. & Mrs. Night Terror work in much the same way. Many nights find me sleeping, albeit haltingly, from sunset to sunrise with no real after-dark surprises. Then there are the nights, where for no reason or cause, that I am dogged *by "scare your pants off"* nightmares that see me kicking and screaming as my wife Sarah tries yet again to call me back, back to where it's safe, back to a wakeful state. As unpredictable as where a summer shower may hit. PTSD certainly does keep me on my toes, that's for certain.

Happily, there is always something to be grateful for. I have long been a "glass half full" person, so finding gratitude is never very far from the surface.

If I shine the searchlight back over the last few years, daytimes are easier. Like the Gold Medalist Olympic dancers who have worked for years on perfecting their dance routines, so have I learned to dance with my brain injury. Unlike Olympians who spend time apart, my dance partner and I are forever together. We know each other - and there is a sense of comfort in the familiar.

I have to stretch a bit further with my PTSD. The less-than-friendly nights are fewer than they were a year ago. And a year ago, they were fewer than the year prior. Looking back, I can see progress. So when I look forward now, I have hope. I have real hope that next year will be easier than this, and that the year after will be easier still.

And it's largely because of that hope that I am able to get up every day, and move, however slowly, forward in my new life.

Getting Back on the Bike

"I learned that courage was not the absence of fear, but the triumph over it."
~Nelson Mandela

There was never any question about getting back on a bike after my accident. Not riding would have been like not breathing.

"So David, do you plan on breathing again now that your accident is behind you?" Silly questions are just that - silly.

When a teenage driver, barely old enough to shave, careens into you at 35 MPH, damage is done. Bones break, tendons tear and brain injuries come to pass. And when the battle lines are drawn between a cyclist and a few thousand pounds of speeding metal and glass, the cyclist rarely wins.

But I survived. We aren't called *"survivors"* by chance.

For the first few months after my accident, I was relegated to the basement on a stationary cycle. I watched way too much Dr. Phil as I spun for an hour or so every day. Driven by some urge deep within me,

I kept up my daily exercise regime and waited for my bones to mend.

And the day finally came. I ventured back onto the streets of my town.

Learning to live in a body powered by a damaged brain takes time, lots of time. And so it was for me for those first few months. I didn't know what I didn't know.

Putting on my cycling clothes started the adrenaline engines. I was pumped up before I ever left my driveway. Cruising through my neighborhood felt great. I was still so innocent, still so new to all this "TBI stuff." I was going to beat this - or so I thought.

And then it happened. I came to a road with a solid yellow line, two lines of traffic in front of me. I froze in my seat.

I'd like to share that I crossed that road and continued my ride, but such was not the case. I carried a secret that even I didn't fully understand at that time. My PTSD was now calling the shots.

And it spoke to me quite loudly at that intersection. "Thou Shall Not Pass!"

It took me over six months to be able to cross a street with a yellow line, so ingrained was my abject terror of anything metal and fast-moving. But time passed as it inevitably does and slow-by-inch my world got larger.

Fast forward to today.

I cycle twenty to twenty or more miles most every day. It's been a couple of years since I felt "yellow line terror." Yearly I take a short ride from our home in Southern New Hampshire to drop by my mom and dad's house. It's really not that short at 100 miles. Not bad for a middle aged, brain damaged guy.

A few months after my accident, a member of the medical community shared with me that pumping highly oxygenated blood through a damaged brain speeds healing. While that alone is motivating, there are so many more reasons to stay in the saddle. By cycling most every day, I am taking an active role in my own recovery.

I am one of the fortunate ones. When TBI brain fog and unfathomable mental exhaustion mean that time at work is done, I can still hop on my bike and ride for a couple hours. My tired brain has a chance to rest and recharge a bit as I leave those things that exhaust me - things like phone calls, conversions, email and the like are left in the dust.

And pretty consistently, somewhere around the fifteen mile mark, gratitude washes over me. It may be something as simple as passing a few cows, or cycling through a pine grove, my senses awakened.

Living with a traumatic brain injury is the toughest road I never expected to walk.

But I'm doing it - one mile at a time.

The Journey Continues

*"The Road goes ever on and on
Down from the door where it began.
Now far ahead the Road has gone,
And I must follow, if I can..."*
~J.R.R. Tolkien

It was on day much like yesterday that part of me died; a cold and blustery typical November day with steel cold bright sunshine that brings no warmth. Trees more barren than colorful, an austere visual reminder that winter will soon knock on our door.

Never one to really plan my daily cycle ride, I passed the place where grit, glass, metal and my flesh collided almost two years ago. I pass this same spot a few times a week with little or no emotion.

Not so yesterday.

Fast approaching the spot of my near-death, the wind picked up and sent earthbound leaves spiraling skyward in a colorful fall tornado.

And I wondered...

On the level or pure energy, were fractured pieces of my own soul still part of the unseen landscape?

Was part of who I used to be swirling skyward?

Earth and soul.

Seen mingling with unseen.

Remnants of my fractured Soul swirling skyward telling me it's time to let go, to move on. To continue my rebirth and reinvention?

Counting down the last few days until the two year anniversary of my accident. And I know with every fiber of my being that it's time to let go.

To give up the ghost.

To let my past life slip away.

To try to embrace the changes.

To accept that I am living my Second Life.

But letting go is hard. Perhaps the most difficult thing I have ever had to do.

Perhaps it's time.

But my past has claw marks on it.

And yet again, the lyrics that have been part of our lives for so many years define reality.

"I'm shell shocked from some heavy blows

A stranger to the people I know

Who used to say "he never had a down day"

Now I'm holding on to can't let goes

And silence brings no peace..."

~Another Life, Third Eye Blind

Yeah, I'm holding on to can't let goes.

Life has taken on such a level of surrealism. Two weeks ago, a reporter from New Hampshire's largest newspaper sat in my kitchen interviewing me for an upcoming story about my recent book release. We spoke again this morning.

And what I heard shocked even me.

She was in an auto accident during Hurricane Sandy. And, like me, she sustained a significant head injury.

"David, so much of our interview and your book came back to me while I was in the ambulance. You will never know how much it helped me."

Is it my Fate to join the national emerging narrative about TBI? What are the chances that a reporter covering a book about life after brain injury has her own mere days after our interview?

Going to do the best I can to ride out this week. At this time next week, I'll be starting Year Three.

Can it get any stranger?

I need to go tighten my seat belt for the ride of my life.

"I am Disabled."

"The first step toward change is awareness. The second step is acceptance."
~Nathaniel Branden

I spit out three simple words with about the same degree of dignity that a cat yacks up a hairball.

It was an unexpected admission that brought about unexpected emotion.

Just about every brain injury survivor I know defines life by "before and after." We count the days, months and years since both "births." We are born into this world originally and we start lives anew as brain injury survivors.

I am 52 years old and three-and-a-half as well. If you are a brain injury survivor, you know exactly how this feels.

And so it is for Sarah and me. In our lives "before," we were frequent travelers. But brain injury has a way of making life smaller - much smaller.

Tough decisions had to be made during that abysmally tough first year or so after my traumatic brain injury. As my ability to earn a living continues to be compromised, we had to sell my Jeep. The monthly payment, easily made before my accident, soon became the cause for a monthly panic attack.

Hello traumatic brain injury, goodbye Jeep!

No longer is there a sense of sadness about this as material "things" come and go. I've learned that pain comes from holding on to things I'm supposed to let go of.

Like a Jeep Wrangler... or my old life.

In our "old lives," we were more than occasional travelers. But alas, said that Winnie-the-Pooh narrator who offers the running monologue in my head these days, all that is in the Previous Chapter in the book of our lives.

Which now brings us back full-circle to being disabled.

Sarah and I recently took a trip. Though nowhere near as frequently as we did in our past loves, we are still fortunate to be able to occasionally get out of Dodge.

While trying to set up seat assignments, the US Airways online seat selector quickly became my nemesis. Try as I might, I was unable to find side-by-side seats for Sarah and me.

I need to be painfully honest here... this once confident traveler was more than a little frightened by the thought of sitting alone for a couple of flights.

In fact, I was scared witless.

Over time, as life with a brain injury becomes more familiar, I am ever so slowly getting just a bit more comfortable asking for help. This gradual acceptance of my new limitations has come to me at a snail's pace, but it has come.

And I made a simple decision to call the airline.

A sincere and compassionate representative named Susan took my call.

"I am disabled," were the first three words I spoke.

I shared my challenge of being unable to sit with my wife. And I openly shared that I am a traumatic brain injury survivor.

Five minutes later, this angel in human form not only has Sarah by my side for our flights, she moved us closer to the front of the plane with a few magical mouse clicks.

"That will make things easier for you, Mr. Grant. Is there anything else I can do to help you?" compassion clear in every spoken word.

Tears welled in my eyes and my voice was shaking as I humbly thanked her.

Brain injury recovery does not happen alone.

Once I found a whole world of other survivors, it was close to a cake-walk to reach into the TBI community and ask for help. I find it harder, much harder in fact, to reach outside my comfort zone and identify myself as brain injury survivor to the World at Large.

It's hard, it's humbling and as I've learned, sometimes it's necessary.

By far, the toughest part of my journey, the darkest time of my entire life, in fact, was the time before I met other survivors... when I walked the TBI path alone.

But I've learned that there are people along the way, some part of the brain injury community and others who are simple kind members of our shared human family, who are happy to help us find our way.

Learning to Walk

Hi God, it's me, David

"When the solution is simple, God is answering."
~Albert Einstein

I know I should check-in more often. We both know things can get busy. I only have a handful of kids and that keeps me busy enough. I can't imagine having a few billion Children to look after.

Thanks for understanding. God knows my heart is in the right place. Um... yes, You know.

I'm still working on healing. It's been such a long road. It's been a bit over 28 months since the accident that came close to ending this leg of my soul's journey. Sarah and I are both happy I'm still here. Stuff gets hard sometimes. Living life since my accident has been such a trip. Sometimes I feel like I "do" less but like I "am" more. It's hard to describe. I feel like a deeper thinker than I ever was.

Being so near to death probably does that to a lot of your Kids.

Take today, for instance. I pushed out 15 miles on my mountain bike. I wear an old sock over my neon green cast to keep the road dirt off it...and to cause passers-by to not do a bit of a double take.

And today I thought about stardust.

Since my accident, I've taken up an interest in nuclear physics. That alone is a bit of an oddity. Most of your Kids don't realize that all the matter that we see, all that we touch, all that defines the word as we see it, all that matter comes from exploding stars. Every atom and molecule that makes me is a piece of stardust. Virtually every human being who has walked the Earth since time began is made of stardust. It's a bit humbling.

Can I ask you a question?

When I look into the night sky and see stars, am I really looking at the building blocks of people yet to be born? The raw ingredients of souls yet to be born? There is so much mystery in Your world.

I'm going to do my best to keep on healing. So much has changed since my brain injury. It's like the very foundation of my world has shifted. What's up is down, what was left is now right. There was a time in my past where I placed a bit more value on the material than I should have. But if I look at the richest of the rich in today's troubled world, all that material wealth will not add a single heartbeat to someone's life.

Ahhh, but You've shown me that by trying to give back, the number of my heartbeats may not increase, but the value of my days is beyond that of the richest of men. In Your infinite wisdom, You have granted me that and so many other new awareness's.

For those gifts, I thank You.

I'll try to not get so busy that I sometimes forget to say thank you. But please know that in my heart, in my heart of hearts, I am grateful that you spared my life 28 months ago.

And if I really believe that You spared my life, I know it was spared for a reason.

A reason I am still trying to figure out.

I guess that makes me pretty human.

Developing Compensatory Strategies That Work!

"However beautiful the strategy, you should occasionally look at the results."
~Winston Churchill

So much of life when we are younger is centered on the process of learning. We learn to speak. We take those cumbersome first steps as we become toddlers. Fast forward a few years as we learn life skills, like reading and writing, which enable us to become a productive part of society.

Our "learning journey" continues as the years pass as we learn to drive, and learn skills through education that we will need in adulthood.

For most people, once a specific skill set is learned, they move on through life. But traumatic brain injury is a veritable game-changer. Like an eraser on a super-sized pencil, traumatic brain injury can virtually erase so much of what took for granted.

This I can share from a personal perspective for it was on November 11, 2010 that a giant eraser in the form of a TBI "erased" much of my life. It was on that fated day that a teenage driver broadsided me while I was out on my daily 30 mile cycle ride.

In two ticks of a clock, my life was forever changed.

While many folks who have sustained a TBI know immediately that "something was different," such was not the case for me. Symptoms of my brain injury started to surface slowly over the first couple of months after my accident.

In the second month after my TBI, my ability to speak was abruptly compromised. For someone who communicates for a living, this was a devastating blow. Unending vertigo struck with equal force making the simple act of walking an unexpected challenge. As memory issues surfaced, my ability to remember the day of the week, or even the current month began to evaporate.

Like a giant eraser cutting a swath through the middle of my life, my traumatic brain injury was erasing, sometimes quickly, sometimes slowly, the skills I needed for daily life.

If the story ended there, this would be a tragic tale indeed. But such was not the case. Long before my TBI, I was known to be quite tenacious. Sometimes even called stubborn. Looking back with the benefit of a bit of hindsight, it was my stubbornness that saved my life.

I simply was not going to let my brain injury beat me. We only get one shot at this life. If my fate was to be a brain injury survivor, I was going to make the most of it. From my strong-willed standpoint, there were no other options.

Slowly, over the months that followed, I did my best to try to understand what my specific new deficiencies were. It was only after they were both identified and understood that I could start to develop new compensatory strategies to again live my life.

A few of my TBI symptoms self-resolved over time. Gradually, at what felt like a snail's pace, I watched vertigo drift further into the background of my life. As I was also diagnosed the Post Traumatic Stress Disorder, symptoms well beyond my brain injury haunted me as well. It was well over two years after my accident that my persistent PTSD nightmares stated to abate.

But many of my new found challenges simply would not go away. The passage of time proved to not always be my friend.

For example, when it became clear that my ability to be certain of the day of the week was not coming back, and that my recall of the current month was not getting better, it became time to look at an alternative method for enhancing my compromised ability to recall.

This took the form of a multifunction wrist watch with the day, date, month and year within arm's reach. Though this may sound like a natural solution to my chronological challenges, brain injury sometimes hides such simple solutions from me.

"It can't be as easy as just wearing a different watch," my mind shouted out when my wife Sarah suggested this solution.

My mind was wrong and Sarah was right!

To this day, when I have the need to quickly pull the day of the week out of my hat, I no longer rely on my brain. Rather, my instinctive reaction is to look at my watch. I did not relearn how to pull this information from a damaged brain, but found a new way to achieve the same result.

A year into my life as a traumatic brain injury survivor, I went on a fact-finding mission in the form of neuropsychological testing. I needed an impartial, highly trained individual to help me to best identify those areas that were still deficient. As my testing wound down, the neuropsychologist made what I now know to be a life-changing suggestion.

"Move as much mental processing out of your brain as possible." He went on to share that this would free up my remaining internal resources for the tasks of day-to-day living. Suffice to say, he was correct.

From moving my ability to tell time to the outside of my brain, to using a web-based calendar to schedule they day-to-day events that defined my life, slowly, over many months, I slowly migrated into a new way of living.

Yes, that eraser wiped away so much of my life. At first, I thought this to be a bad thing. But now I see it for what it was. By cleaning the slate, I was able to being much of my life anew.

I read a while ago that traumatic brain injury is the last thing you thing about, until it's the only thing you think about. While this is true, I have found that a new life, one very much worth living, can be rebuilt.

Developing a new way to live my life has become close to second nature to me. While it does not take away that fact that much of my life is more challenging than it's ever been, it does leave me open to trying new solutions to unexpected TBI related challenges. Suggestions that now have a proven track record of improving the quality of my life.

An Unexpected TBI Teaching Moment

"Life is a long lesson in humility."
~James M. Barrie

In late 2010, my life was forever changed. It was on a cold and blustery November day that the unthinkable happened.

As an endurance cyclist averaging 30 miles a day at the time, I took great pride in my untainted cycling record. Logging over 50,000 miles on my trusty bike since 2007, my cycling practices were very much on the conservative side. Obeying traffic laws, using hand signals and the ever-present neon yellow jacket helped keep me safe.

Safe that is, until a teenage driver broadsided me and catapulted me into the new world of traumatic brain injury.

Now well into year three since my TBI, I still marvel at how little mainstream America knows or understands about traumatic brain injury. With 1.7 million Americans sustaining a TBI annually, it is the elephant in the living room that no one wants to acknowledge.

As life moves forward, as it inevitably does, I find myself in a new role- that of being a TBI advocate. Never one to shy away from the opportunity to be of service to others before my accident, using my new life's experience has provided me with countless opportunities to share about traumatic brain injury.

Even now, years later, life still presents countless TBI "teaching moments."

Never expected, events unfold in such a way that often provide unique ways to teach others about traumatic brain injury. And sometimes the tables are turned in ways that are nothing short of profoundly stunning.

Such was the case this past February, on the 27 month anniversary of my TBI. I was the teacher in this unexpected opportunity. And the student, you might be wondering?

A young doctor.

Some things you just can't make up. Truth is so often stranger than fiction.

And so my journey continues...

I was recently injured in a cycling accident of a much smaller magnitude than the one that caused my traumatic brain injury. As I have continued cycling, about the only inconvenience in New England winters is a bit of snow. Being more tenacious than anything, I wait it out, and when the roads are dry again, I'm back at it.

The comments of a medical professional a few months ago strengthen my commitment to wellness. He shared that highly oxygenated blood pumping through my brain is healing and that there is hard data to prove this.

But a sudden February snow squall and a patch of black ice brought me down hard. There is no such thing as falling gracefully. Falls are hard. They are ugly. And they can be damaging, quite damaging.

Circling the wagons back to my TBI teaching moment, I found myself sitting in an exam room with the same orthopedist I saw right after my 2010 accident.

As he examined my still sore hands from my accident, we engaged in a little time-passing conversation.

"Yes, the weather is looking up."

"Not too much longer till spring."

You know the type of light chatter to pass the time. He asked me how I was faring since my 2010 crash. And I let him know he was cited in my book. He is the orthopedist that predicted my broken arm would take six months to heal. And he was spot on.

Sizing him up, something in my soul let me know it was time to drop the bomb.

"I was left with a traumatic brain injury as a result of being struck by the car in 2010."

He stopped his careful manipulation of my hands, took a deep breath and just looked at me for a minute or so.

And he dropped a bomb of his own.

"You don't look like you had a brain injury."

We know the five words that define our new normal...Not all disabilities are visible.

What was my reaction?

So, doc, what am I supposed to look like?

Not even close. I seized this teaching moment to teach the good doctor a bit about TBI. I talked. Openly. Honestly. Candidly.

And much to my delight, he listened. Not a courtesy type of listen, but he heard me. And he learned. I was able to again advocate for traumatic brain injury survivors. A member of the medical community now has a much deeper insight into the quiet world of TBI.

I am grateful. Profoundly grateful. As a younger doctor, if fate is kind to him, he will have decades of treating patients. And if someone comes to him and is a member of our most exclusive TBI club, he will be better able to offer compassionate care.

Seen in this light, though painful, my fall might just be worth it. Others will now benefit by receiving care by a doctor who now better understands that looking "normal" is not an indicator of a brain injury.

After all, anyone familiar with the challenges faced in living life with a TBI well understands that looks can be very deceiving.

Traveling at the Speed of Light

"Time travel is such a magic concept."
~Matt Smith

If there's anything I've learned since my traumatic brain injury, it's that life is not always fair.

My wife Sarah and I were still relative newlyweds when the hand of Fate struck hard. We had just celebrated our one year wedding anniversary in August of 2010. A few months later we began our new lives. Mine as a brain injury survivor and Sarah's as a survivor's spouse.

If you asked what changed since my brain injury, one word sums it up: everything.

Over the years since my brain injury, I've learned to laugh again. If you had shared this with me at most any time during that abysmally tough first year, you would have been met with disbelief.

I was incapable of seeing through the brain fog and unable to envision, even remotely, a life worth living. If you are still early on, trying to regain your footing after a brain injury, hold on for quite a ride. But know this - it will get easier. I was told this by folks during my tougher times and quite frankly, I didn't believe it. I believe it now.

Life as I knew it and life as Sarah knew it ended abruptly on a cold November day. Little did we know, however, that a new life was beginning for us.

Over time, new compensatory strategies began to emerge. From embracing technology to manage my time to simply realizing that some things are just not worth worrying about, life has gotten easier.

Where I used to have good hours, I now have occasional good days. Where there was nothing but darkness, fear and no real hope of living a meaningful life, there is now an acceptance that life is different, but okay. And there are times I know a peace that I never knew before my injury. Go figure. I never saw that coming.

Sure, life is a bit slower, but it certainly didn't stop.

Almost five years ago, Sarah and I honeymooned at Disney World. We had such fun on our honeymoon that we decided to take a honeymoon every year. These plans were laid down before my accident. Thankfully, we are able to continue our tradition.

And it's at times like these that there are some things I have come to really appreciate about having a brain injury. So much of this new life has challenges, so why not embrace a few odd quirks of life after brain injury?

This year, our Honeymoon will take us from our home state of New Hampshire to Montana to Glacier National Park. From door-to-door, it's over 2,500 miles.

Here's where it gets fun.

Since my brain injury, I am no longer able to discern the passage of time. Perhaps you are in that club as well. In the spirit of complete disclosure, there are times I love it. A three hour flight to Florida "feels" more like 25 minutes.

"Ladies and Gentlemen, this is your Captain speaking. If you have had a TBI, prepare for a very short flight. The rest of you - well, make yourself comfortable for the next few hours."

Or those occasional trips we take to visit my Mom and Dad in the northern part of New Hampshire. It takes Sarah two hours to drive there. Me? Our ride north "feels" like twenty minutes.

The blessing of time travel has a downside. There are two sides to every coin. I can return a call from a friend that I thought was a speedy reply only to be told that it took me two weeks - or more - to do something as simple as returning a phone call. Those who know me, who really know me, take it all in stride.

Sometimes I am embarrassed. Most of the time, however, I just chalk it up as part of my new life and move on.

It all feels a bit like science fiction. Like I am living in some endless loop of the Twilight Zone. I can't explain why my ability to discern the passage of time is gone.

This summer, if you happen to be on a flight to Salt Lake City and see someone in seat 11B with a bit of an awkward smile, it might just be me enjoying travelling at the speed of light.

Reclaiming Intimacy

"Intimacy is something to be cherished."
~Ira Sachs

It was one of those quiet moments just before we both drifted off to sleep. The kind of quiet talk that almost never leaves the bedroom.

"No one ever seems to write about challenges with intimacy after a brain injury," I said, sleepily.

"Then do it," said Sarah. Her voice had a degree of conviction that almost kept me awake.

Almost.

Talking about love, sex, and intimacy can be like unraveling a tangled web, even to those without a brain injury. Add a brain injury to the mix and these difficult to discuss subjects can look insurmountable.

Prior to my traumatic brain injury, Sarah and I were equals in every sense of the word. In fact, those who knew us before my brain injury often called us one of the most happily married couples they had met.

One of my fondest memories of life "before" was a question we used to get four, five, six or more times a year: "Are you two newlyweds?" Sarah and I have long been fond of living an immersive, present life. We have always loved to travel. And before my brain injury, we had more than a decade of walking through our days, hand in hand, experiencing so much that the world has to offer.

Always holding hands — her hand fits most perfectly inside mine, we apparently have the look of a couple of people who really like each other. So, up would come that question again: "Are you two newlyweds?" We'd walk into someplace small, quaint, and intimate. It might be asked at the Pink Pig Café in Sedona, or perhaps that little coffee shop on the edge of Moab, Utah, just outside of Arches National Park. I've lost count of how many times in 15 years that a random stranger pops us that question.

Such is the outward manifestation of the love we share inwardly. We are blessed to have found each other. Even more blessed to know what we have.

I share this so you can get a bit of a real-feel for who we were before my brain injury.

Professionally, I was a web developer and a blossoming writer. Sarah has a career in telecommunications. We were two successful, very independent people who found great joy in just being us.

You already know what's coming next.

Then "it" happened. The driver who broadsided me while I was cycling was only a child of 16.

And our life — all that we knew, all that was familiar, all that was intimate — was torn from us in two ticks of a clock in a mangled wreck of steel and broken glass.

A large part of the David that Sarah knew, the David that Sarah fell in love with, the David that Sarah married ... a large part of who "he" was and who was one half of "us" no longer existed.

From an equal, I became her ward. I was under her guardianship. And for a time, our status as equals was gone.

Relationships without a brain injury are complex enough. Add a brain injury to the mix and most everything is unpredictable.

Intimacy is most natural when two people love each other, body, mind, and soul.

Many years ago, I heard sex defined as "an outward manifestation of inner love." It's a definition I have come to love.

But brain injury is an intimacy game changer. The first dynamic affected comes from changing roles. During that first year, I became dependent on Sarah for so much. She became my caregiver, making sure that I took care of myself, ate, rested, and set limits based on my new disability. The list goes on.

To be able to simply jump into our old roles as equals after the lights went out was simply not possible. Mental exhaustion leads to physical weariness, which in turn leads to instant sleep when head hits pillow. Hardly a recipe for intimacy.

Add the complexity of changed relationships, and it's easy to see why many marriages don't survive the pressures of a brain injury.

At one point, Sarah dropped a bomb. She said, "If we didn't have as many years together as we did, we probably would not have made it."

But made it we did. Thankfully, the hardest times are behind us.

Everything about me has changed. Yes, I look the same. I know you understand that. But under the hood, everything is quite different. I react more openly to life. I laugh more than I ever have. I cry at just about anything. I am a different husband, partner, lover, and hand-holder than I was before.

But, I know, too, that at the core of me, deep inside of me, I am still, and always will be, David.
 Thankfully, Sarah sees and understands this, often even more than I do myself. She has the ability to see through my brain injury and see the person with whom she originally fell in love.

Life today is similar but so different.

We still hold hands most everywhere we go. Not because of some sense of obligation. Rather, it's because we feel close with even a small bit of physical contact.

And those who know us as a couple, who really know us, know that it's not been easy. But they see that love covers a lot of ground. And they see the look we have in our eyes as we gaze at each other.

Slowly, we are rebuilding a new "us" on the same foundation that worked the first time: mutual respect and a deep love for each other. We have found that open, sometimes raw, occasionally awkward conversations about love, sex, and intimacy are critical in helping us come to understand, embrace, and live in the "new normal" of our relationship.

Nothing beats the realization that you can get through just about anything with your best friend by your side. And at night, when all is quiet ... well, we'll just leave it at that.

Learning to Live in the Moment

"Write it on your heart that every day is the best day in the year."
— Ralph Waldo Emerson

In hindsight, it's probably best that we didn't know what was coming. No one really wants to know that life is about to become difficult - very difficult.

It took several months for the severity of my own TBI to become clear. Early on, well respected doctors - doctors doing the best they could in this strange and so often unpredictable land of traumatic brain injury - predicted a complete recovery.

A few weeks after my cycling accident, one of my first neurologists shared that I "would be back to 100% within a few short months." Always one to rise to a challenge, this didn't bother me a bit.

As time marched forward, his timeline for my complete recovery changed a bit. Months passed and I still had significant "issues." He upped the ante a bit and let me know it might be three years, but certainly no longer than five years, until I fully recovered. I would be completely normal again.

Looking back on this time with the benefit of years behind me, I see now that the good doctor really was doing the best he could. I have no room for lingering resentment or animosity as these are barriers to forward progress. Life can be challenging enough.

There really was such innocence during that first year after my accident. Sarah and I thought we were just biding time, waiting for life to return to normal. Life did return to normal, but it's the new TBI normal. We'll circle back to that later.

There was so much we just didn't know during year one post-accident. I find myself unexpectedly grateful for what we didn't know.

We didn't know that even now, well into year four, those PTSD nightmares would still haunt me. We didn't know that there really is no end game in brain injury recovery. We didn't know about the friends we would lose, the financial hardships that were coming; that life as we knew it was coming to a close.

Nine months after my accident, Sarah and I travelled to the Florida Keys. We were still living in the "Age of Innocence" as we were both expecting me to recover fully. A week in the balmy tropics seemed like a near-perfect way to help speed along my recovery. We basked under a mid-summer's sun, hopped from tropical beach to tropical beach, did lots of hand holding and figured we were still on the right track as my recovery continued.

Had we known what was barreling toward us at light speed, our trip would have been filled with dread and fear. Now precious memories would never have been made.

Over three years have passed since our first trip to the Keys. This past summer found us back in the Keys again, a bit older and a whole lot wiser.

We have both learned so much along the way. The most meaningful life lessons come from living through what life puts on your plate. No longer does Sarah or I pay much attention to predictions. Trying to predict brain injury recovery is like trying to put a saddle on a cat. You can try really hard, but in the end, it becomes nothing more than a lesson in frustration.

More importantly, living life "in the moment" has become one of the biggest forward moving steps we have taken. The past cannot be changed. It's a cancelled check. The future never really comes. It's a promissory note.

This past summer found us walking on many of the same beaches that we walked on a few short months after my injury. Thought the beaches were the same, I am different now.

During our most recent trip, we passed a small nature trail at Bahia Honda State Park. In the Summer of Innocence back in 2011, Sarah and I walked a nature trail there. Both shutterbugs, she and I, we snapped countless flora and fauna shots. One of those butterflies travelled north with us in digital format. Never would I have imagined that this winged beauty would be the exact same butterfly I would use on the cover art for my book.

Tears filled my eyes as we passed that same trail. It's been such a long journey. Sarah never even turned to look at me. She felt high and sudden emotion rise from deep within me. Her grip tightened ever so slightly. We are connected at a soul-level like that.

Yes, living life in the moment is the real key to being OK with all this. In the moment, there is no fear of an uncertain future. In the moment, there is no regret for choices that could have been made differently. There is safety, security and peace to be found in this moment.

And at least for now, in this exact moment in time, I am OK with that.

Developing a Meaningful Life

"Our prime purpose in this life is to help others."
~Dalai Lama

Life is so often unpredictable. Many years ago, my dad shared with me an interesting thought. "If I had the opportunity to see the future in a crystal ball, I would most likely pass on the opportunity."

I was younger and thought his comment to be pure folly. Today I see the wisdom of his words. Given the same opportunity, I can now say that I would pass on such an opportunity as well.

On November 11, 2010, the course of my life was forever altered. Not a gradual changing of life's direction. No, fate had something a bit different in store.

It was on that fated day that I was struck by a teenage driver while I was cycling and catapulted into the new, strange and often unpredictable world of traumatic brain injury. No one asks for a brain injury. A brain injury is just about the last thing you think about, until it becomes the only thing you think about.

I was rushed by ambulance to the nearest trauma center, my wife Sarah following the speeding ambulance in her car. A local police officer appeared at the trauma center to take my statement in case it was my fate to succumb from my injuries.

Over the weeks that followed, the extent of my brain injury became clearer. My new normal included a speech challenges including aphasia and stuttering. Memory challenges became almost comical, and PTSD with its symphony of symptoms became my constant companion. We can add to that incessant tinnitus and a good case of vertigo that robbed me of the ability to walk straight.

The first year of my life as a traumatic brain injury survivor was the hardest year of my entire life.

At one year after my accident, I knew it was time to get as well as I could. Though everything I had read spoke to the fact that brain injury recovery was lifelong, I harbored a secret that perhaps I was going to be different. I was going to be that one in a million who came back from a brain injury as if I had never been hurt.

As time passed, it became clear that I was in for a marathon and not a sprint. My attitude shifted. No longer was I hoping to "beat" my brain injury. My goal changed to learning to "coexist" with my disability. That goal exists to this day.

My first step in this process was to learn more about exactly how I was compromised. By getting a real feel for what was in need of repair, I could better move toward a new wellness.

There are a few benefits to having to cover medical costs out of pocket. When it became time to find a competent neuropsychologist, I was able to do so based on input from other members of the TBI community. I was not relegated to finding an "in network" or insurance approved doctor. I had the freedom to choose based on proficiency alone.

At the conclusion of my neuropsychological testing, my wife and I had a final meeting with a trusted doctor who "got it" regarding brain injury. So many of the sections of testing found me scoring at the bottom of the scale that the doctor let me know that I was permanently disabled. The insight that his testing offered was invaluable.

Looking back now with the benefit of a couple of years of hindsight, he was no doubt correct. At the time of my testing, one year after my brain injury, I was disabled. But that was just a snapshot of how I was at that time in my recovery, and as we know, recovery is indeed lifelong. Neural plasticity is an amazing thing.

I took my newfound information and started to formulate a recovery plan. One of my biggest decisions was to change my attitude. Never will you hear me say that I "suffered a brain injury." Never will

I have the attitude that I was the "victim" of a cycling accident. Words like "suffering" and "victim" are mental and emotional barriers to moving forward in life. They restrict my forward movement.

The reality is this: if you have a heartbeat, you've had unpleasant events come to pass in your life. Children get sick, parents age, jobs are lost, and cyclists occasionally get struck. Part of the human condition is that life unfolds for all of us. I am not exempt, nor are you. The bigger question was this: what was I going to do to make the most of the rest of my life?

My mind was quickly made up. Though I might never get back to 100%, I became a bit driven to get back as close to that as possible.

Like snowflakes, every brain injury is different. There is no "one size fits all" treatment protocol. Rather than looking at my brain injury as a single challenge, I opted to look at my injury as a series of individual symptoms. In essence, I broke it down to a much simpler form.

I was not just someone who had sustained a brain injury. I was a person who was trying to find an effective methodology to live with tinnitus, a person who was trying to find a way to live with a memory that so often failed me. I was a person who was trying to relearn to speak with a speech impediment. While learning to live under the enormous weight of a brain injury may seem overwhelming, learning to find compensatory skills for individual challenges was much easier.

I made the decision to take smaller bites out of the apple. And it's been a game-changer. In fact, there are times there is almost an element of fun to it all. That is a far cry from where I was a few months out, thinking that life as I knew it was over.

In my book, *Metamorphosis, Surviving Brain Injury*, I chronicle the trial and error in developing new compensatory strategies. For example, my initial solution to my memory challenges was to try to use those yellow sticky notes seen everywhere. Being a bit of a tech guy who happens to have pathetic handwriting, I opted for a 21st century approach by using digital sticky notes on my PC. Some models have flaws and so did this one.

Sticky notes are only good if you read them. One day, a full month after I decided to use the sticky note methodology, something on my PC caught my eye. Looking closely, I saw that I had not even looked at my notes for weeks. Sitting right in front of me were scheduled tasks, all uncompleted, gathering digital dust. So much for digital sticky notes!

As memory problems remain challenging, I needed to find a new method for moving as much of my memory outside of my brain as possible. As a long-time user of Google's calendar feature, when I saw that I could sync my Android phone to my calendar, it was close to the end-game for many of my memory challenges. It became second nature for me to add life events to my calendar. Unlike my hidden PC sticky notes, every time I turn my phone on, my reminders are in my hand and are now rarely forgotten. Of course, if Google goes out of business, I am in deep trouble, but it's doubtful that will ever happen.

Symptom by symptom, solutions began to present. None of these eliminated my deficiencies. Rather, they became compensatory strategies allowing me to coexist with my new shortcomings.

While many of these strategies are unseen by most, there are a couple of cases where others benefit from my new strategic approach to life.

Virtually every day since November 11, 2010, accident-induced tinnitus has robbed me of any real silence. But I have a life to live, said the voice in my head that so often sounds like the narrator in a Winnie the Pooh tale. I am a believer that we all must be the biggest advocates of our own health care.

Now that the memory challenges were at least becoming more manageable, it was time to find a work-around to offset the ever present ear ringing that was robbing me of any peace. In the summer, we stay cool with air conditioning. Moving from one cool oasis to another, we find respite for discomfort. Akin to air conditioning, I have developed a compensatory strategy that I fondly call "Ear Conditioning."

My office is "ear conditioned" with a fish tank on my desk and a robust aerator pushing bubbles that my desk-bound fish frolic in. It drowns out the constant ringing.

Our bedroom is "ear conditioned" as well with a white noise machine on my dresser. While I have choices like waves, rain forest sound and more, I opt for the soft chirp of summer crickets at night—blotting out the constant tinnitus.

As PTSD has made our world smaller, the last couple of years have found my wife Sarah and I spending more time at home. Since my accident, new grape trellises adorn our landscape, flowers of all varieties blanket our yard. And a new love, aquascapes, has allowed me to bring "ear conditioning" to our yard. By our back patio sits a fishpond with a waterfall, the soft gurgle of our backyard stream a welcome distraction. I installed that one the first year after my brain injury. I've come to find that water gardens and their accompanying relief are like chips: you can't have just one.

Year two found me adding a small reflecting pool, spitting frog and all. Yes, a bit more auditory bliss from that one. And just this past summer, I got "the itch" again and added a nice fountain to our back deck. You no doubt see where I am going with this.

Those who don't know my condition (as I look quite normal) see it as a wondrous landscape. But me? It's a coping strategy helping me to live a meaningful life with a brain injury. The fact that I happen to create wonderful waterscapes is... well... just the icing on the cake.

In the three years since my accident, life is slowly taking on new form. Over time, acceptance replaces fear. Finding compensatory strategies that work build confidence. And life, though vastly different than life before my brain injury, becomes again worthwhile.

So much of my life these days involves advocating for those whose life has been impacted by a brain injury. While nothing can take away the challenges that come with trying to rebuild a life after brain injury, knowing that others have been helped by the experiences I've had makes this new life a life of real and meaningful purpose. And for that, I am grateful.

No Two Paths are Alike

"A life is not important except in the impact it has on other lives."
~Jackie Robinson

My Fate has lead me down a path where I do have a very unique insight into the realm of brain injury that only comes from living it. If you add together every bit of knowledge I've gleaned from the books I read, the websites I've poured through, the doctors I've talked to, the summation of all of that "outside information" is only a speck of dust compared to what I've learned firsthand by actually living daily with a brain injury.

One of the great revelations in all of this is that no two paths are alike. My brain, unlike any other part of me that might, over the course of my lifetime been injured, takes its own time to recover. Its timeline is completely its own.

My greatest single period of recovery thus far was at the fifteen to sixteen month point after my accident. At that point, I walked through a period of recovery that was both unexpected and profoundly life-changing. For the first time since my accident, I have moments - moments mind you - of life that was close to normal. I had glimpses of my pre-accident self. It was akin to being reacquainted with an old friend.

No, there was not the absence of all challenges. But it was like the volume was turned down on many of my most glaring symptoms.

If you are reading this and are a brain injury survivor who has been told you are as good as you'll get, I implore you to not pay attention to what you were told. I am glad I chose not to accept what I was told and continued my aggressive road to recovery well beyond the one year point.

At one of my monthly brain injury support group meetings, a member shared that year three was her year of the most gains.

Yes, every journey is different. My experience is part of my own personal journey, and you have your own path to walk. But pay limited attention to those who share information that may hold you back.

The TBI Zone

"It may be said with a degree of assurance that not everything that meets the eye is as it appears."
~Rod Serling

So often I have heard from others, souls who have others close to them living with a TBI. The comments always move me deeply.

"You have helped me better understand what my (son/daughter/mother/father/husband/wife) is going through."

Brain injury knows no boundaries.

With Sarah out of town, I find myself writing a bit more. I hope you don't mind. If you've read this far, you most likely don't mind.

Things are about to get strange, really strange. Twilight Zone strange. You are traveling through another dimension, a dimension not only of sight and sound but of mind. A journey into a wondrous land whose boundaries are that of imagination.

Your next stop, the TBI Zone!

Living daily with a brain injury defies logic and defies explanation. A whole new set of nonsensical rules apply. Sure, there are quirks and oddities that I never expected. I can no longer feel the sensation of being cold. I never liked the cold anyway so there's no real loss there.

And those who know me know that I would run from seafood as if it was the plague. I ran away from all things aquatic for close to a half century. Not anymore. Truth be told, I have enjoyed catching up on decades of crab. In fact, these days, Sarah and I have a seafood night once a week or so.

I count down the days every week until Crab Fest Night, only to begin counting again. Such is the power of my new found love of crustaceans.

But it's the memory changes that are the most surreal. I wrote about this at length in my book, Metamorphosis, Surviving Brain Injury. In my book, I compared my memories to snowflakes in a glass snow globe.

DJ drove into me at 35 – 40 MPH in 2010 and shook up my globe, each flake a memory. Memories long buried came to the surface. I could recall one conversation from 1971 like it was just yesterday.

Creepy.

(🎵 🎵 *Insert a bit of Twilight Zone music here.* 🎵 🎵)

In my first life, I had a pretty normal memory. I fondly call it a "linear memory." I could look back in my life and see that an event happened last week, last month, or even a few years ago. It was pretty much the status quo for anyone uninjured. It was a garden variety memory.

After my brain injury, everything changed. My memory became flat. Instead of looking at events in a liner timeline, events in the past are like sticky notes on a wall. In my mind's eye, I "see" the memories, but can no longer tell you when events came to pass.

Yeah, weird.

Last week I was at a bit of a get-together at a local college with a number of friends. Looking across the room, I saw Jerry. My first thought was that it was nice to see him as it has been a couple months since our paths crossed last. If recall serves me correctly, we had coffee together on a couple of occasions.

Trekking through the crowd, I gave him a hearty, "Great to see you again, Jerry."

He looked at me a bit askance and dropped the bomb.

"Yeah, I've not been here in nineteen years."

Bombs like this no longer surprise me. As time passes and I now better understand my own post-TBI limitations, I got better at just rolling with things. Better to roll than stand slack-jawed looking silly.

Nineteen years.

In my mind's eye, it was a few months ago. I real time, it was close to two decades. We chatted for a couple minutes and bomb 2.0 came.

"What was your name again?" he asked me quite innocently.

(♪ ♪ How about just a bit more Twilight Zone Music for effect here? ♪ ♪)

I let him know again that it was good to see him again and never mentioned my brain injury. After all, I still look normal, though twenty years older to my old friend Jerry, but still normal all the same.

Driving home from Merrimack College, I was lost in my thoughts thinking about how much life had gone down in close to two decades. A divorce, the birth of one of my sons, a move to a new town, then another, then another. A career change, then another, and another. Marrying my Soul mate, the list goes on.

These days, when Sarah and I talk, I don't usually reference linear time. This I learned the hard way by referencing something that happened last week, only to be reminded that it was a year ago... or more.

"Sarah, remember in the past when...."

Using a generic reference to the past is a compensatory strategy. Does it bother me? This lack of ability to not realize when things happened? Not really. It adds just another layer of surrealism to life.

Just what I need.... more surrealism!

Watching Out for Rogue Waves

"It is better to err on the side of daring than the side of caution."
~Alvin Toffler

Occasionally, rogue waves make the news here in New England. For those unfamiliar with rogue waves, they are solitary creatures, spawned many miles offshore. They roll in catching unsuspecting sea-goers by surprise. Not your average wave, these enormous waves have been known to wash innocent souls out to sea.

They come out of nowhere, crash our shorelines and recede as quickly as they rise. They are simply part of life for anyone with coastal roots.

And just like seaborne waves can wreak havoc, so can the emotional waves that come with living as a brain injury survivor. Like their aquatic counterparts, they originate out of nowhere, offer a bit of emotional catastrophic damage, then recede, sometimes as quickly as they came.

As the four-year anniversary of my traumatic brain injury nears, an emotional rogue wave has come close to swamping my boat. And like those caught unaware at the seashore, I have been caught completely off-guard.

The last couple of weeks, I have seen a huge resurgence in the overwhelming sense of loss and grief. Shared before, my hope was to be that one-in-a-million person who completely recovered from a brain injury. For so many years, my "plan" was to wake up one day, wipe the sleep out of my eyes, and like magic I would be who I was before my brain injury—whoever that was.

Ever so slowly, I am letting go of that secret hope. Sometimes, I am okay with the fact that this is my life and that I have to make the most of it. At other times, the dark thoughts come back. The rogue wave that has crashed over me tries to pull me under.

During the first year of my new life as a survivor, a therapist saved my life. She made me promise that if I ever considered looking for a "fast pass" to the finish line of life, I would call her first. "If I suspect that you are going to harm yourself, you know what I have to do," she said with the civility of a drill sergeant. At that point in my life, a locked psychiatric ward with mo doorknobs and the removal of my shoe laces held no real appeal.

Feeling the weight of it all, this past week I Googled, *"brain injury and suicide."* No, I have no intention of cashing in my chips. Rather, I was more than a bit curious about how many others died from traumatic brain injury long after the initial injury. The numbers were staggering.

My new life these days is defined by living close to complete transparency. I share more than most ever will, knowing that my own complete disclosure will help others to feel less alone and less isolated. As my wife Sarah has shared since life forever changed in November of 2010, "the curse will become a blessing."

The process of evolving from one person to another almost completely different person is often hard to describe to those who have not lived it. But it is a process. There will be good days, and there will be tough days. On the tough days, it helps to remind myself that I have a 100% track record of success in making it through the tougher days.

And that rogue emotional wave that came crashing down? Unlike solo beachcombers, I don't have to ride that treacherous wave alone. In the years that have passed since my traumatic brain injury, I have met so many others who have successfully navigated the unfamiliar waters of life after brain injury. Their support and success gives me hope that I can find a way, however haltingly, to live this second life I now have.

If today is one of "those days," where the wave looks too big, too much to handle, too overwhelming, try to remember that you are not as alone as you might think. Others are there to help you find your way.

TBI Injustices

"One must never forget that life is unfair. But sometimes, with a bit of luck, this works in your favor."
~Peter Mayle

Sitting across from my dad last Sunday at a local eatery, he shared something that caught my ear. "The principal of our elementary school was just fired," he said as casually as if talking about the weather.

He went on to say that she had a recent skiing accident, hit her head, and was having trouble with her memory. Student's names now escaped her. Teachers she had known and work with daily were also among the unremembered. And the town took action; action in the form of termination.

There are so many layers to this short story. If her TBI rendered her incapable of executing her day-to-day functions as a school administrator, what other options did the local officials have? A leave of absence? More medical care? As I was only privy to a small snippet of the story, these well may have been presented to her.

But the take-away is this: yet another life forever changed by traumatic brain injury.

The numbers are staggering. By the time the sun sets today, another 5,000 join this exclusive TBI club. And 5,000 more tomorrow, and the day after...and the day after, ad infinitum.

The challenge for so many of us is that we lose our voice, our clarity at the time we need it most. It's hard to self-advocate when you are in early recovery from a traumatic brain injury.

In my case, I was on my trusty bike when I was struck by a teenage motorist. Some of you know that already. What you may not know is this: the insurance company that represented the driver denied all claims. When they concluded their investigation, they deemed me to be 51% at fault. When I asked the representative if the investigator was a neutral party, I was told that the accident investigator was on the insurance company's payroll.

Have a great day, Mr. Grant. Thank you for contacting our insurance agency.

I was dumbfounded. Thousands of dollars of medical debt, and the loss of earnings that will impact me for the rest of my life.

Have a great day?

A couple of respected local attorneys were contacted. As my accident was of the "right of way" variety, I was told they are difficult cases to win.

Have a great day, Mr. Grant.

Was I bitter? Yeah, bitter is an understatement.

But time passed as it inevitably does, said the narrator voice inside my head, sounding a bit too much like the voice of a Winnie the Pooh narrator.

Over time, perspectives change.

When Sarah and I were left essentially on our own, the realization came quickly: sink or swim.

So I started swimming.... merely treading water at first, with waves of live and heath challenges crashing over my head.

BUT I KEPT SWIMMING.

Over time, the swimming became a bit easier. Not easy, mind you, but easier. The waves that crashed over my head were a bit smaller.

It was well into year two that I paid off the last of my medical debt. That alone is a blessing. It felt like I had paid off a mortgage.

I will continue to swim. If you are a survivor, you well know that none of this is easy. Yes, there are bright spots, but there is a dark side as well. A side where nothing short of oblivion looks like an option.

There is so much injustice served to those who can't speak for themselves, whose brain fog and new life limitations mean no clarity of thought or action. And my thinner emotional filter means just thinking about it moves me to tears. So many of my new friends have been railroaded by insurance companies and more.

No easy answers, no quick cure, just a snapshot from inside the mind of a TBI survivor.

What about you? Was "the system" fair to you? This question alone might ignite a firestorm.

But to speak of our pain, our hardships, our injustices lets others know they are not alone.

We find strength in each other and carry each other. I will carry you as so many of you have carried me.

Life is like that.

Let's Talk About Fear

"Thinking will not overcome fear but action will."
~W. Clement Stone

Let's talk about something so many of us can relate to. No pussy-footing around.

You know that little four-letter word none of like to admit lurks just beneath the surface.

Let's talk about... FEAR.

Many who know me, who see an occasional picture of my wife Sarah and I smiling for the camera... many might be tempted to think that I have all my ducks in a row. Yup, you might even think that my crayon box is full, and that all my clowns are happily at my own circus. You might even think I'm zero cents short of a dollar and that my elevator never gets stuck between floors.

Sorry to shatter the illusion kids, but I have more challenges than most ever know.

These days, I have a new breed of friends – internet friends. While I have no shortage of real human friends, I have a few folks who I have yet to meet.

Like me, Mike Strand had his writing published in last year's Chicken Soup for the Soul book about traumatic brain injury. Though we have never met face-to-face, he feels like a brother from a different mother.

Mike eloquently notes, "I am pretty high functioning and most of the time I can keep my brain injury from being the most noticeable thing about me."

That is me to a tee.

Say "hi" to me at the store or cross paths with me along this road of life and you might just think I am normal and uncompromised.

But after a few short minutes, you'll see that I really am missing a couple of crayons in my box.

Sarah and I are just back from a few days off. Vacations are good for us.

But vacations are harder and quite fewer since my injury. It is what it is. She worries about me, watches over me... and our pace is decidedly slower.

In a quiet moment this past week, I shared a secret fear I have. No longer do I even know if it's the first time I've told her. My injury has robbed me of the ability to recall conversations past – making me at times feel like Dory in Finding Nemo.

"Boo, sometimes I get scared when we spend a lot of time together," I said with a bit of apprehension. "I'm afraid that when you spend more time with me, you'll see how screwed up I really am," I confided.

Her reply was not what I expected.

"I already know how screwed up you are," she said with an easy smile that let me know immediately that it was said with unconditional love.

And in two ticks of a clock, the illusion was shattered. I "thought" I did a pretty good job of looking like I was okay, and that my deficiencies might not be as noticeable as I thought.

We are going to graduate from a four-letter word to a five-letter word.

I was WRONG, dead wrong. I wasn't fooling anyone, except maybe me.

Here we are, well into year five and I am still learning more about how my day-to-day life is impacted by my injury. It's like peeling skin of an onion – under ever layer is yet another layer.

And fear came surging back. Yeah, I told you we were going to talk about fear. It was only a matter of time until I circled back to fear – but you already knew that.

Fears abound... What will our future hold? Some studies show long-term risks of other health challenges after a TBI.

Will my kids ever come back in my life? The scorecard as of today: three of my four sons have elected to walk out of my life. If I think about this one too long, it paralyzes me.

We said "for better or for worse," but that irrational voice in my head tells me that she didn't sign up for this. I have lost a lot, but I still have enough left to know that this is so hard on her. I forget so much while Sarah remembers every bit of it... every good day and every tough day.

Last week, I wrapped up my taxes. Me and effective time-management are not friends, but that is a tale for another time.

Last year was yet another year of declining income. Too much information? I don't really care. I know I'm not alone in this one. Our financial future is a scary place, so I try not to go there. For many years, I was the breadwinner – a term I find archaic and antiquated – but it will have to suffice until something new comes along. This has now changed.

A few months ago (or it may have been a couple of years ago) I shared this fear with Sarah. The what-if-we-can-no-longer-afford-our-home fear.

She asked me what a worse-case scenario was. "A small apartment," I shared.

"In your irrational fear, will I be with you?" She asked, knowing the answer already.

"Yes, "I said somewhat sheepishly.

"As long as we are together, I'm okay with whatever happens with our lives," she said.

Everyone should have their own Sarah. Mine is already spoken for.

But this new life, this TBI life... it can be a scary place to be. There is so much uncertainty. Yes, uncertainly is part of the human condition, but a TBI tends to magnify things quite a bit.

Someone wiser than me once said that F.E.A.R. stand for False Evidence Appearing Real.

I can only hope. And for now, that is really all I can do – hope. I can hope that in the end, all will be OK. I need hope as much as anyone.

Yeah, I may look normal... but now you know the rest of the story.

Dead Man Walking

"No one is so brave that he is not disturbed by something unexpected."
~Julius Caesar

They looked at me like they had just seen a ghost.

And in one respect, they had.

Just prior to the three year anniversary of my traumatic brain injury, I stopped by my local service station to get my yearly vehicle inspection sticker. We are kind of funny about that here in New Hampshire as we like vehicles that cruise our highways and by-ways to be safe. Better for you, better for me.

Doing not much more than killing time as my car was being inspected with surgical precision, my eyes drifted to the intersection directly in front of me. Cars passed back and forth, an occasional truck passed by and I waited patiently for the technician to finish his task at hand.

And in two ticks of a clock reality struck me like a stick.

I was staring at the very intersection where I was struck by a teenage driver just shy of three years prior.

For a moment in time that seemed to stretch for longer than it should have, I wondered how I found myself at that exact spot without giving much thought to it.

In one respect, that fact alone shows me that I am ever-so-slowly healing.

A couple of minutes later, as I was paying at the counter for a new inspection sticker, I asked the attendant a couple of simple questions.

"Have you been working here for a while?"

The gentleman, a retired school teacher, shared that this was his 'retirement job' and had been for six years.

And I had to ask...

"Do you remember a cycling accident right out front a few years ago?"

And I waited. My heart was pounding in my chest.

His eyes had that far-away look as he mentally walked back through time.

"I'll never forget it. It was horrible. The guy on the bike was hit right there," he shared, pointing to the corner.

"And he flew head over teakettle all the way to there," this time pointing to a spot 40-50 feet down the road.

He went on to tell his version of the day Fate intervened in my life, about how the local fire department closed Main Street, about all the first responders who walked from the fire station a mere block away to attended to my broken body.

And I dropped the bomb.

"I was that guy."

Four simple words.

He looked at me like I was a dead man walking.

"It was a horrible accident," he said again as he sized me up with new eyes. As expected, he then asked me how I was doing these days.

Rather than using this as a TBI teaching moment, I opted for the easier, softer path.

"I've still got stuff, but I'm alive."

As I was leaving, he called over to the station owner.

"Remember that bike accident a few years back? He was 'that guy' who was hit."

"Such a horrible accident," echoed the owner staring at me like I was supposed to be dead.

I smiled, cordially thanked them both for taking care of my car, and walked, legs shaking, back to my car.

Thankfully, the PTSD is getting easier, the nightmares less frequent. I was unexpectedly grateful to simply be alive. To have a heartbeat. To still be able to hold my wife Sarah's hand. Just "to be."

Seeing the accident that caused my traumatic brain injury through the eyes of others was quite surrealistic.

But then again, so much of my life today as a brain injury survivor borders on the surreal.

And if your life has been touched by traumatic brain injury, you are no doubt nodding.

Because like me, you get it.

Learning to Soar

To Infinity & Beyond!

"This isn't flying, this is falling with style!"
~ Buzz Lightyear

Buzz Lightyear, the now infamous space ranger from the Intergalactic Alliance, has quickly become my TBI hero.

Let's hop in the Wayback Machine, shall we? And go back... back into deep space-time before my brain injury.

Back to a time when I was unaware of all the new acronyms that now define my new life.

Back before TBI.

Back before PTSD.

Back before MRI's, EEG's and ABI's.

Back when I still lived in blissful innocence as to what my future would hold. To when life was easier and care-free.

Sarah and I have long been fans of Disney World. Both Sarah and the Magic Kingdom were born in 1971, so there is an element of cosmic Karma to it all.

For many years, the four seasons were defined as spring, summer, fall and Disney. Being ostensible Disney fans, we learned the art of travelling affordably many years ago.

In our life before brain injury, a couple of trips to Disney every winter were not uncommon. Like kids at Christmastime, we'd count down the days until our trip from MHT to MCO in ever-building excitement.

And the Disney parks... let's just say that we know them like the back of our hands. Where to go first, how to play the Fast Pass game, where to get a frozen latte. It was a familiar routine we cherished in our life "before."

So much so that when we planned our honeymoon a few short years ago, only one destination made the list. Like so many other mouse-ear clad newlyweds, we spent the first week of our married life playing like the kids we really are.

Life was good. Life was innocent. And while not perfect, life was easy. We had each other. And no idea what the future held in store.

We were married for just over a year when I was broadsided by a teenage driver. We had fifteen short months of married life before my brain injury. So much of life with a brain injury is unfair. Sarah has been married longer to the "new" David then she was to me before my accident.

That alone makes me want to stamp my feet and pout... and cry foul.

But to what end?

We all get what we get. There really is no Wayback Machine, except on TV.

On a recent trip to Disney, I let Sarah know that I wanted to take a vacation from my brain injury - that I wanted to play like we used to. That we needed a vacation from life.

And play we did - for five long days.

And I came home broken. Ruined. Exhausted.

It was a month or so until I had recovered. But that is a tale for some other time.

But I has the opportunity to see Buzz Lightyear again. Buzz has long been a Superhero to me. Since my brain injury, my fondness for Buzz has increased tenfold.

We saw him last December at one of the character meet n' greets. There were 20-30 small children in line to see him. My feet stopped abruptly and my mouth fell open. To this day, I regret not getting in line.

I watched innocent child after innocent child hold out an autograph book and pose for a quick picture.

Sarah watched my reaction and encouraged me to get in line.

But I was embarrassed. These days, I care less about what the world thinks. But not so on that day.

So what it is that I love about Buzz?

Stay with me on this, OK?

Buzz believes he can do ANYTHING. We all know his wings are plastic, but he BELIEVES he can fly. Even his best friend Woody tells him he can't fly.

Best friends are like that – the support each other unconditionally. I am blessed to be married to my best friend. She believes I can fly.

You see, Buzz has blind faith. Faith that anything is possible- despite unseen limitations.

He believes in miracles. And in the Power that dwells within him.

And so I play connect-the dots with my own life; my life since my traumatic brain injury.

There have been people in my own life who have told me things could not be done.

A neurologist who said I was permanently disabled.

But, like Buzz, I chose not to believe the limitations that were placed on me by others.

Like Buzz, I choose to fly.

Having my emotional filter all but torn from me is not always bad. As I sit here typing, tears run down my face.

Tears of gratitude.

I have many role models. Some have heartbeats, while others have batteries.

And I also have dreams. If you happened to be in the Gamma Quadrant of Sector 4, and see Buzz, keep an eye out for me.

You see, no one ever said I could get there. But more importantly, no one ever said I couldn't.

And if I lose my way, I recall Buzz's sage words...

"This isn't flying, this is falling with style!"

A Brain Injury Milestone

"Life is a journey and it's about growing and changing and coming to terms with who and what you are and loving who and what you are."
~Kelly McGillis

Last Saturday night, I climbed exhausted into bed a few minutes before Sarah. Two back-to-back nights of PTSD nightmares and little sleep left me bone-weary with emotions on high. And I was only a few hours away from the two year anniversary of the day that has left me forever changed.

It didn't take much. She wrapped her arm around me like she does every night and I burst immediately into sobs, my mind racing with all that has come to past in two short/long years.

"Have you asked for help?" she whispered softly.

There was no way I was in the mood to do ANY business with God. How could Anyone let one of his own kids go through the tormented existence of what life can be like with a brain injury? Nope. Not only was I not talking to God last night, I was talking to no one. Exhaustion magnifies things. Sadness is greater, intolerance creeps in unasked for. And hope dwindles.

She lay next to me, whispering softly to me as I cried. My tears slowly turned to sleep. What she said, I cannot say. But I am grateful to have her love.

And I slept like only the dead are capable of. And awoke to my two year anniversary. And my sleep was a game-changer.

By 11:00 AM, I was home from my daily 30 mile cycle ride, my Victory Ride.

Lots of thinking, of reflecting... and memories unbidden.

In the trauma center, I slipped away. Strapped to the back-board as the extent of my injuries were being evaluated, I did a little trick.

Now you see me, now you don't.

Like being pulled backwards through a long hall, reality was fading fast. I could watch events in the ER, but it was like looking through a long telescope through the vastness of space and time. Everything distant, diminished... dimmed.

And Sarah called me back.

"David.... David...."

I can recall the look of terror in her eyes as she looked down upon me, my eyes open and staring straight ahead, blank, glassy and empty. She knew I was gone.

Yet she called me back.

It was only a few months later, in a counseling session, that I was told by a medical professional this was a typical near death experience. Did Sarah pull me back from deaths door? My own personal jury is still out on that one, though I am inclined to believe that she did.

The last two years have been the toughest of my life. But it's OK.

I gave lots of thought today to my own recovery. To pieces of my old life that I have been able to pick up.

Since my accident, I have recovered most of my ability to speak. Just the other day, Sarah said I no longer stutter, that I now just stammer. While this may sound like a small victory to some, it's huge to me. I love the art of communication. To be able to articulate my thoughts in a way that makes you think, to expand your own horizons, to ponder what you never gave thought to. To have a large portion of that stripped from me was painful.

Over the last couple of years, I have made 24 on-time mortgage payments. A year ago, I was not sure if I would be able to keep the gears of life turning. Time has shown that, while the gears occasionally grind, they are still in motion. I am grateful for that.

My experience laid the groundwork for my latest book, Metamorphosis, Surviving Brain Injury, written entirely after my accident. No small feat for a man labeled by a respected neurologist as "permanently disabled."

At Mile 15 on my ride today, I had an epiphany. That happens more often than I ever expected. Clarity emerging from sweat.

It was the Hand of God that caught me when I was hit. Yes, you heard me. The teenage driver who hit me was cruising along somewhere near 40 MPH. And he never hit his brakes. There are so many ways this all could have unfolded- all of them with me passing from this life. I could have been hit by a truck. A larger car could have been my Fate.

But no. It was a small subcompact car with a low bumper and a gently curved hood. The bumper hit my leg and I rolled up the hood into the Safety Glass windshield. This simple acrobatic act absorbed enough of the force of Impact so as to keep me alive. Not unbroken, mind you, but alive. And I thank God that my life was spared. Countless others who sustained the same type of trauma have passed from this life, yet I live on. How can I not be grateful?

Sarah and I spend most of the day yesterday putting our yard to sleep. Leaved were raked, branches were trimmed and beds were cleaned out for a final time. Yet one rose remained in our back garden. Once I finish today's writing, I'm heading out to cut it.

We are heading out shortly to one of our favorite walking places today. Perhaps an end of the season picnic, perhaps not.

But the rose is going with us.

We have a stop to make along the way.

The trip to the park means we pass by the exact spot where two years ago today, life forever changed. We are stopping at that spot to place the single rose there. I shared this with Sarah today and she just smiled.

It's time to let go of who I was and embrace my new life.

And it's only fitting that the rose we leave today was grown by Sarah's gentle touch...

Life after Brain Injury - I Have a Secret

"Limits, like fears, are often illusions."
~Michael Jordan

I have a secret.

Not all is as it appears. Most anyone living with a traumatic brain injury already knows this.

All I have to do is tell you, "You look normal." At this point, you will either want to bop me on the head, or you'll simply shake yours and think, he just doesn't get it.

But I do get it. I live in the new 'Frontier Land' that is life with a brain injury.

A chance meeting with a neighbor let me know that I am not the only one with a secret.

About a year after my brain injury, a new walker appeared in my neighborhood. Not a zombie walker like those in the Walking Dead. No, this was a man a bit older than me. One day he appeared with a cane and his wife, ever present by his side.

As I still cycle twenty-five miles a day, I know most all of the neighborhood regulars by sight. I have given most odd-ball nicknames like 'Dog Walking Lady,'

'The Power Walking Couple' and more. Here was a new player on the Stage of Life.

My wife Sarah and I drove past these walking souls regularly. Month-by-month, you could see his pace increasing and his stability improve. "I bet he had a brain injury," Sarah prophesied.

Quite unexpectedly, I found myself stopped at a corner on my bike as they walked by one day.

The disinhibitionism that comes with brain injury can be so freeing.

My first words brought huge smiles to them both.

"You are doing so well. It's GREAT to see the progress you've made." Introductions were shared, though his name, like so many others, is forever lost to me.

And the conversation flowed like water.

He fell on ice the year after my TBI and joined our exclusive brain injury club that no one really wants to join. Brain injury is indeed the last thing you ever think about - until it's the only thing you think about.

"The doctors said I would never get any better, but I decided not to listen to them," he chuckled. I listened intently to his tale for 5-10 minutes and smiled.

Then I dropped my own verbal bomb. "My brain injury was a year before yours and like you, my own doctor said I was permanently disabled and to not expect much. I didn't listen either!"

We shared a hale and hearty laugh and went on our respective ways.

And my secret?

My TBI has taught me that all is not as it appears.

That man fumbling with his wallet in front of me at the checkout counter no longer causes impatience.

He might be someone affected by traumatic brain injury

That driver cruising along at 10 MPH under the posted speed limit no longer makes me tap my foot.

She might be one of the 3.5 million people affected by brain injury this year.

The person at the supermarket with his buggy parked dead center of the aisle as he stares at all the soups?

You know where I am going with this. We are everywhere.

My TBI continues to teach me a level of patience, understanding and compassion I never had before my accident.

When someone passes by you wherever life happens to take you, remember that they might just be one of us.

After all, we look normal.

Developing Effective Adaptive Strategies

"Learning never exhausts the mind."
~Leonardo da Vinci

Over the years, more than a few people have said that I ought to give serious thought to a career as a photographer. While I am flattered by the kind words, I'll never even consider it. But the reason for this resolute decision might just surprise you.

While I have partially recovered from my 2010 cycling accident, there are still so many lingering challenges that I face as a brain injury survivor. My "visible" injuries have healed as they should have. My bones mended, my bruises faded, my lacerations healed.

There are no lingering physical challenges whatever. In fact, if I were to head to a physician unfamiliar with my history, I would emerge with flying colors, a specimen of fine health. This, of course, provided that I never said the three words that have forever changed me: Traumatic Brain Injury.

Rather it is my "invisible" injury that stubbornly won't let go. As time passes and I learn more about the medical aspects of being a brain injury survivor, I realize that I really am simply a typical TBI survivor.

Yes, every brain injury is different, but there seem to be some common threads, some shared traits that we, as survivors, have come to live with.

I tire more easily than I used to. In my case, it's a metal fatigue that can wear me down in ways unlike anything I ever dealt with in my life "before." My emotions are closer to the surface than ever as well. If you are a survivor, you most likely understand that feeling.

But of all the challenges I now face, my compromised memory is, without question, the biggest challenge of this new post-TBI life. I'm not talking about the "where did I leave my keys?" type of occasional challenge that most everyone faces. If it were just that, life would be so much easier.

There are days now that my memory fails close to 100%. Events that passed a month ago, feel like last week. Occasionally I'll reference something in conversation with my wife Sarah thinking that it was a relatively recent occurrence - only to be told that I was talking about an event from a year ago - or even longer.

It's hard on me as it rocks my confidence and self-esteem. It's even harder on those closest to me as it's an "in your face" reminder that I am not as well as I look.

But like so many other challenges I face as I walk this new path, all is not lost. Not even close.

And so we circle back to my incessant picture taking.

After a year or so as a brain injury survivor, I went through extensive neuropsychological testing. Said a trusted neuropsychologist, "move as much of your mental processing to outside your brain as possible."

My cloud-based calendar helps keep my day-to-day schedule in order. And my picture taking helps me to find order in a past that would otherwise be jumbled and meaningless. At least once a week, I transfer images from my calendar to my external flash drive. These "digital memories" are sorted in folders based on dates.

They are my bionic memory! I can easily go back digitally through time and see what happened last week, last month, and even last year. All the guesswork is gone. Most of the frustration is gone. Sure, there can be an extra step in recalling events that have come to pass, but it so worth it.

And realistically what options do I really have? I can continue to experience frustration. That is always an option. But I chose to listen to my doctor - to try something that is perhaps a bit non-mainstream.

But in the final analysis, it works. And isn't that all that really matters?

Living an Unfiltered Life

"All faults may be forgiven of him who has perfect candor."
~Walt Whitman

Some things you just can't see coming – like a traumatic brain injury. Never did I envision the life that I have today. It's only natural to look forward in your life when you are younger. Some people yearn to become doctors, race car drivers, or even astronauts, but no one wants to grow up to be a brain injury survivor.

Brain injury is the last thing you think about, until it's the only thing you think about. And so it was for our family. At forty-nine years old, my professional career was in full swing. I had just married the girl of my dreams. There was a healthy and fun rhythm to our lives, days were long and the sun shined upon us.

Until that fated day in 2010 when everything changed. And I do mean everything.

For many who share our fate as a survivor family, they remember "the call" or the knock on the door. If you live a life defined by traumatic brain injury, you most likely have memories of "that day." Perhaps there was a car crash or a fall. Domestic abuse brings some into this new TBI life. There are seemingly endless causes with one shared result – a traumatic brain injury.

Learning to live with a brain injury is a bit like learning to drive a new car. The controls are off a bit. Everything that was familiar is now unfamiliar. It takes time to get used to the new normal of life after TBI. In my case, it took many years.

And the changes... so unexpected, so surreal. However, not everything that defines the new normal of life after brain injury is a bad thing.

For example, since my own brain injury, I've developed an instant love for seafood. I spent close to half a century avoiding all things aquatic that end up on a dinner plate. No longer! Truth-be-told, my new life has become a bit of a Food Channel type of adventure. A recent trip to Louisiana found me sampling local fare like crawdads and frog legs – something that never would have come to pass in my old life. I find the new culinary adventures quite wonderful. My wife Sarah doesn't seem to mind.

Changes in my tastes and personality transcend just about every aspect of my life. Today I live an unfiltered life as my brain injury has essentially wiped away my emotional and verbal filters. No longer does anyone say, "So David, can you tell me how you really feel?

These days, I am learning, often the hard way, to say less. My emotional and sometimes verbal filter departs at the most inopportune of times.

"Mr. Spock, the shields are down, increase verbal output to warp factor five."

Get in front of me in the twelve items of less aisle in the grocery store with thirteen (or more) items in your basket and you might just see me behind you in line struggling to call you out on it. This alone is growth. In my first year or so as a survivor, there was no struggle as I'd simply call you out on it.

But the loss of my emotional filter has proven to be one of my hidden TBI Blessings. I can freely and without worry or concern share what's on my mind. Better still, I seem to be able to put the brakes on when I need to, when tact or decorum are required. It's not uncommon now for me to tell my aging dad that I love him. The first few times he heard me say that, you could hear a bit of awkwardness creep in, but no longer. We are both new Englanders and have been trained for generations not to wear emotions in public. No longer. I can thank my brain injury for this new freedom.

I openly and often let those close to me know that I appreciate their presence in my life. If I have an opinion, I generally share it these days. Those close to me know that subtlety not part of the new David.

Time passes and my old life seems like that of someone else, memories that dwell within me belong to someone who once was. Such is the everlasting surrealism and unending reality of life after TBI.

But today, just today mind you… today that is okay.

Where There's Life, There's Hope

"Everything that is done in the world is done by hope."
~Martin Luther

To say that traumatic brain injury complicates relationships is an understatement of monumental proportion. Brain injury affects more than just the actual survivor. Husbands, wives, children and parents all feel its effects. Friends slowly fade away as life forever changes.

With what might be called a more "traditional injury," time passes and everyone involved moves on with their respective lives. Not so with a traumatic brain injury. The after-effects last a lifetime.

My own brain injury occurred just over four years ago when a teenage driver struck me while I was cycling on a mid-November day. As the years passed I knew the collateral damage was high, but there are some things you just can't see coming.

My oldest two sons were in their mid-twenties when our lives changed forever. One was a web developer, the other looking to pursue a career in criminal justice. They were the types of kids that any parent would be proud of. Though much of what I read during the first couple of years after my accident talked about fractured friendships and families, I was quite sure my life would be different.

A bit over four years out and my naiveté shines bright. Both of my oldest boys are nearing thirty now. And both have made the decision to fade into the background of my life. One faded away in 2011, the other a year or so after my injury.

Brain injury? Yeah, it's complicated. As I started the abysmally slow and painful crawl toward my new normal during my first year as a survivor, I heard the whispers.

"Dad is faking that brain injury stuff for attention," came the silent voices that I was not supposed to hear. Internet research was done and I was labeled by several family members as having a mental disorder in which a person fakes illness to gain attention and sympathy.

In what amounts to a cruel twist of fate, these accusations came at a time that I was least able to advocate for myself. I was doing all I could to understand where my old life went. Barely having the internal resources to live my new life as a brain injury survivor, the option of having the option to what amounted to defending myself was not even on the table. The lack of my reply to accusations only fueled the rumors that my injury was indeed being faked.

As time passed and the absence of my sons became acute, the lack of return calls, the deleting of email and the non-responsiveness to text messages made it clear that they chose to believe the rumors.

Time passes as it inevitably does, said the Winnie the Pooh narrator voice that so often describes the timeline of my life. Earlier this year, after many years of failed attempts, I surrendered my sons to the Universe. Oh, how I would love to share that this was a freeing experience, that my hours of prayer paid off and that a joyful reconciliation came to pass.

But they are still AWOL.

Last month I deleted my sons' numbers from my cell phone. It was painful and moved me to tears again. Just when I thought the river of tears had dried up, the waterworks started. I did not delete them for reasons you might expect. Daily, when I would use my phone, if my contact list happened to stop on an "S" or a "D," I'd again see my sons' names on my screen. And in seeing their names, the pain would often come rushing back with a vengeance. Little did I realize that the toughest part of my post-brain injury journey would have come to this, but such is the reality of life after brain injury.

Those who know me best, those who really know me, know that my default setting leans decidedly toward optimism and having a positive outlook. These two attributes have carried me far in this second life. So what type of positive take-away can come of this?

I've learned that family is not defined by shared DNA. There are people who are part of my new family who love me unconditionally. I am grateful to have so many souls like this as part of my life. And I cling to the old adage that says, *"Where there's life, there's hope."* In spite of how things have unfolded over the last few years, my not-so-secret hope is that my sons will eventually come back into my life.

Brain injury is complicated. More complicated than anything I've ever experienced. But the Beatles were right. I'll get by with a little help from my friends.

To Share or Not to Share

"A man's character may be learned from the adjectives which he habitually uses in conversation."
~Mark Twain

I have so often referred to the first year or so after my own traumatic brain injury as, "TBI Boot Camp." It was undoubtedly the hardest year of my life. Nothing, absolutely nothing in life can prepare you for all that encompasses a brain injury.

The first year or so was painful as lifelong friendships dissolved. It was financially abysmal as my ability to work on a full-time basis stopped rather abruptly when I was struck while cycling, by a teenage driver. My sense of self was as shattered as the windshield that I flew through.

They were tough days indeed.

I talked up my brain injury as if it was as socially acceptable as speaking about the weather. As time passed after my accident, my broken and bruised body did exactly what it was supposed to do - it healed. Well-intentioned friends would ask how my recovery was progressing. My stock answer for much of that first year was about the same. "Other than my traumatic brain injury, things are progressing as well as could be expected," I would share with perhaps a bit too much enthusiasm.

The loss of my emotional and social filter was one of the reasons I found it easy to talk about my brain injury. But sadly, so was naiveté. Don't let anyone kid you. There is still a very real social stigma attached to having a traumatic brain injury. Just ask those souls who used the Opt Out option and quietly faded into the background of my life.

It's been several years since I graduated from TBI Boot Camp. The reality is that I have to live daily in a world where most of those I come in to contact with do not have a TBI. These days, I have adopted much more of a "need to know" approach when sharing. In fact, even the terminology I use has changed.

If I am in a position where my brain injury needs to be talked about, or is even referenced, I use a bit of finesse. Comments like, "I still live with some long-term challenges from a concussion," seem to not alienate others. Unlike the sometimes awkward silence that on more than one occasion has come from calling my brain injury by name, the use of the word 'concussion' seems to be accepted by others much more easily. While 'brain injury' carries a stigma, 'concussion' does not.

This may sound like a small point, but in reality, it is not. I have come to really cherish those relationships that have stood the test of time. I have some loyal friends and family who knew the "old David," and who accept me as I am today. I do what I can to maintain those relationships.

This brings me full-circle to over sharing versus under sharing.

During that first year, not a day went by that I didn't talk about my brain injury. My wife Sarah bore the brunt of my endless TBI monologue. Looking back with the benefit of a bit of clarity that comes only with the passage of time, I needed to talk about it. I needed to work through what was the biggest life change I never expected to happen. I needed the ability to hear myself sort through the chaos and fear. Daily I would talk about vertigo, my incessant ear ringing, the ambiguous grief as I realized I was never going to be who I was before my accident. The list goes on.

And Sarah listened.

Over the years, I have found it unnecessary to continue to share every hill and valley of my day-to-day challenges. This is partially because I have come to accept that this is my life. But also, by speaking of it incessantly, it again becomes front and center, on the stage of our lives.

This past summer, I did what I do most every day - I went out on a twenty-five mile bike ride. But on that particular day, something happened. Occasionally I deal with memory lapses. My damaged brain ceases laying down new memories for a while. On that summer day, I blinked my eyes only to find that I had travelled to a point a half-mile away with virtually no recall.

In what amounts to a sign of post traumatic growth, I regained my bearings, and simply continued along with my ride. It really is amazing what you can learn to live with. I came home, showered and told no one. There was no intent to be evasive. No desire to hide anything. Rather, I chose to not say a word as I just chalked it up to part of what my new life entails.

Over the years since my TBI, I have developed a very strong passion for living transparently when it comes to my brain injury. I often write about many of these events that define my new life. Much of what I write ends up on my blog. And on the day of my amnesia ride, I wrote and posted the story without as much as a second thought. As so often happens, other survivors chimed in that my experience as in virtual lockstep to their own.

Later that week, however, my Dad and I spoke. He shared that he had read of my experience and shared it with my mom. My dad is eighty-one and mom is not far behind. I do all that I can to see that they don't worry about me. I was immediately in that conflicted place of knowing that others need to know that they are not alone and wishing that my dad had not chosen to read that particular piece.

But the real game-changer was when my wife Sarah shared something I had not even considered. "If anything ever happened to you, it's important that I know of anything like this." Suffice to say, she was correct. Life with a brain injury means that I live in a world where things can change in an instant.

Just as I learned that there is tangible effect on others depending on the specific words I use in describing my brain injury, it's equally, if not more so, important that anything that falls into the "big stuff" category is properly discussed.

I continued to learn as I go. Rather than beat myself up for any miss-steps, I'll just call it a learning experience.

Just like recovering from a brain injury is a lifelong experience, so is learning to live life as a brain injury survivor.

Of Fireflies and Thank You's

"A day without sunshine is like, you know, night."
~Steve Martin

Like we have done a few times since my accident, Sarah and I recently made the trip over to the Main Street Fire House here in our small town in southern New Hampshire.

And like every time before, I was barely able to escape before I broke down in tears.

Our last trip there found us bearing a couple of signed copies of my first book, *Metamorphosis, Surviving Brain Injury*. In my book, I chronicled that abysmally tough first year-and-a-half of life after I sustained my traumatic brain injury. As the actions of our local first responders were detailed in my book, it was only natural that they were presented with a couple of copies.

This most recent trip?

A signed pre-release copy of *Chicken Soup for the Soul, Recovering from Traumatic Brain Injuries* was our mutual gift to the first responders who saved my life. This new title features a couple of my stories and was released in June of this year.

Finding the front door to the Fire Station locked, we had to be buzzed in. As Sarah and I shared with these brave souls the reason for our visit, more and more of our local firefighters and paramedics crowed into the small entry room.

"C'mon out back," called out one of Salem's finest as we were led into the main dining area. We've been there before.

You could hear a couple of the guys sharing a few feet away as they ate dinner. "He's the guy who was hit by a car out front."

For those who know might not be familiar with my story, it was only a block from our fire station that I was struck by a teenage driver back in 2010. We met most accidentally indeed in a twisted mess of bent metal and broken glass.

Several of the first responders there that night were on-scene the day I was hit. They spoke of some of the details of that fated day and talked as nonchalantly about my accident as if they were talking about what was going to be on TV tonight.

To them, it was just another accident. To me, the end of life as I knew it.

To call our recent visit 'surreal' would be an understatement.

Inscribed by me, in part, on the inside front cover: *"Thank you for the gift of my life..."*

High emotion surged right under the skin. I struggled to hold it together for just a few minutes longer. Bite the inside of my mouth, look at something on a wall... just don't cry... not yet.

And another piece of the puzzle that my life has become clicked into place.

"My wife now has a traumatic brain injury," shared the Captain on duty as my wife Sarah and I stood there a bit slack-jawed. He was also one of the first responders who scraped my broken and bleeding body off Main Street in 2010.

Since our first meeting, traumatic brain injury is now part of his own life.

"It's been three years," he continued. I quietly did the math. Six months after I became a card-carrying member of this TBI Club, so followed the Captains wife. A head-on car crash caused her traumatic brain injury.

His next two words summed up more than he may realize.

"She struggles."

Don't we all?

"I read your book shortly after her accident," he shared. "It helped me a lot'."

Click. Another piece of the puzzle falls into place.

An invitation was extended to attend our local TBI support group here in town.

As Sarah and I readied to head out for a post-visit walk, another fire fighter asked for my phone number and email address. He asked if I would come speak about traumatic brain injury.

You already know my answer.

Sarah and I were buzzed out following a long round of heartfelt thank you's and warm handshakes. These men are on the front line of life and death. Not every outcome has a reasonably happy ending. Tonight they saw firsthand a life they helped save.

And like it has done since time out of mind, the fire alarm went off at the Station. The heroes I had just spent a few minutes with were back on the truck and heading out to perhaps save another life.

I watched the fire engine come screaming out of the bay. And in the passenger's seat was a man whose hand I had just shaken. He was smiling at us broadly and waving as the fire truck screamed by.

So fitting.

Slow-by-inch, I am healing. It took a good ten minutes for the wave of emotion to crash over me. Fewer tears than last time and more unbridled gratitude.

Sarah and I wound down our night on a local nature trail, most of the nights walk in the dark. The first fireflies of the season were revealed to us, wide-eyed Children of the Universe.

Most of our walk was on the quiet side... Sarah's hand snugly in mine.

I broke our silence with three words.

"I am happy."

Building a Life after Brain Injury, Let's Get Social

"Social media is not about the exploitation of technology but service to community."
~Simon Mainwaring

Traumatic brain injury is a game-changer. For so many living with a brain injury, the world gets smaller. Family dynamics change and life as we knew it is gone.

Brain injury and isolation go hand-in-hand. Personality changes, dwindling finances and a host of other complications can lead to an almost shut-in existence for many survivors. TBI is a family affair that in reality directly impacts anyone even close to the survivor.

As recently as a decade ago, there was no real way for survivors, or those who love them, to connect with each other easily and conveniently. Sure, face-to-face support groups have been around for a very long time. They remain a veritable lifeline for survivors and family members to connect.

But most face-to-face support group meetings are held on a monthly basis. Support group meetings are like an oasis in the midst of a desert, but survivors were relegated to long periods of time with minimal direct contact with each other.

I know this from firsthand experience. My own brain injury was in the fall of 2010. Struck by a teenage driver while out cycling one day, my own life, and the lives of virtually everyone close to me, was uprooted in an instant.

Prior to my own traumatic brain injury, I didn't even have a nodding acquaintance with traumatic brain injury. I never knowingly met one of the several million people who live daily with a brain injury. Any news accounts about the prevalence of brain injury in today's world fell on deaf ears. Somehow I had missed the proverbial memo about the prevalence of brain injury.

I found myself completely and utterly alone after my own injury. For months, I muddled through my day-to-day existence never knowing that there were so many others who shared my fate, others who unknowingly held the key to the end of my isolation.

Several months after my injury, a local rehab hospital started a new brain injury support group. I walked into that first meeting alone and filled with more than a bit of fear. I walked out of the hospital a couple hours later no longer feeling alone, having met for the first time so many others who were... well, just like me. There is a healing, camaraderie, an indescribable bond that happens among survivors.

For the first time, I heard others share about the daily struggles I was living with. Better still, as the years passed and we grew stronger as a group, compensatory strategies were shared and that sense of isolation evaporated - at least for an hour or so a month.

However, in my own life, there was still a void. Weeks without regular contact with others took its toll. In my life before traumatic brain injury, much of my work professionally was internet based. So it came as a surprise to no one that it was to the Internet that I turned again.

No one was more surprised than me to find a vibrant and thriving web-based community of people affected by TBI. From online survivor groups to Facebook groups of all kinds, here were people from around the globe who were communicating with each other on a daily basis.

Gone was the blackout window of weeks between connecting with others who shared my fate. While not quite as intimate as my monthly support group meetings, I was able to connect with so many others with the simple click of a mouse.

I am blessed that my internal compass still points in the positive direction. When living with a brain injury, attitude really is everything. Knowing that a positive outlook can really make life easier as a survivor, I made the decision to jump into the ring. In 2013, I founded what I had envisioned to be a smaller online community - TBI Hope & Inspiration.

My intent was to offer what amounted to a daily positive thought or story about how to live after a brain injury. I underestimated two things: the power of the internet and the soul-level need for other survivors to connect with each other. Within a year, this "small" group blossomed to over ten thousand members from around the world.

Like people, online groups have very unique personalities. Weekly, members ask me to post questions to the group and the response is overwhelming. When a member posts a question about most any aspect of life after brain injury, others chime in to share their own experiences - often within minutes.

And here is where the real miracle begins to take form. So many people living with a TBI have mobility challenges. Many do not drive and many have shared over the years that they don't have access to a local support group. Yet these same people are willing to share their lives as survivors so that others can be helped.

Each member who contributes does so with the intent to help, but comes away from the experience feeling better knowing that they have positively impacted someone's life. Their own heavy load is lightened and they see that their experience as survivors makes them uniquely useful to help others. Their lives are enriched by the very act of giving.

This same spirit can be found in other online groups as well as websites the world over. Living my life as a brain injury survivor remains the toughest challenge of my existence. But when I take a moment to step back and look at how fortunate I am to be able to instantly connect with others, it's difficult not to be grateful.

From a TBI Meltdown Comes New Hope

"Life is very interesting... in the end, some of your greatest pains, become your greatest strengths."
~Drew Barrymore

Sometimes reality taps you on the shoulder with a velvet glove, while at other times reality hits you more like a sledge hammer.

It was on a cold, overcast November day in 2010 that a teenage driver struck me while I was cycling. My bike sustained significant damage. My bike was not the only casualty that day as my brain sustained significant damage as well. There is nothing pretty about being broadsided by a car at 30+ MPH.

Fate could have dealt such a vastly different hand to my wife and me. I looked death in the eye in November of 2010. I could have been just a memory.

A local police officer followed the ambulance that carried my broken body and newly damaged brain to the trauma center on that fated November day. He was dispatched to see if he could possibly get a statement from me, or to be present in the event that I was a pending fatality.

Yes, living with traumatic brain injury is the most difficult path I never knew existed. But it could have been worse... much worse.

Had I died that day, my wife Sarah would have a November anniversary of a different kind. No morbid reflection here, just pondering what could have come to pass.

Several years after my cycling accident, she would most likely still wear the wedding ring I tenderly placed on her finger just a year before the accident. It was only a few months after our first wedding anniversary that our lives forever changed.

Perhaps she would have found a picture of us and wore it in a locket, pulling it out at unexpected times as she felt me reaching for her from the other side, the veil of death separating us for a short time. Memories of things we did, and places we've played would have haunted her for the first couple of years. By year three, those memories might now bring forth a smile, grateful for the time we had together.

Yes, brain injury is a game-changer, but is not the end-game. Life really does go on, even after a traumatic brain injury. Fate spared me a different end to this life. But is also looked kindly on my wife Sarah. We still have each other. Not every relationship can handle the new stress that comes with a brain injury.

As the three year anniversary of my traumatic brain injury approached, high emotion filled the air. The anniversary of my accident was coming at us at light speed. There was a lot of hustle and bustle at our home as the anniversary approached.

And I experienced my first meltdown in a long time. I crashed like a wayward rocket. Uncontrolled emotions drove me to say things I deeply regret. I fell apart in a way I never did in my pre-TBI life. Dragging myself to an early bed, I passed out more from mental exhaustion than really falling asleep.

And I slept like only the dead can sleep. No PTSD nightmares haunted me that night, and I awoke to a new day. Sharing the quiet, still in bed whisper time with Sarah, I commented that the new day meant a fresh start. Her arm around me tightened just a bit in acknowledgement.

Thank God she has a deep capacity for forgiveness. TBI meltdowns don't come often at all these days, but when they come – do I even need to say more? I'm as eligible as anyone.

That very week found me taking to a podium for the first time ever to share my experience as a brain injury survivor as a keynote speaker at a medical conference in Maine. Sarah surprised me with a tie embellished with brains. Rather fitting, don't you think?

I had a unique opportunity to share with so many others what life is like with a traumatic brain injury and to share my very real message that life can indeed be rebuilt after a TBI. Yes, I was excited. But just under the excitement was fear. I still have significant speaking challenges even years after my accident. When stressed or overtired, I can stutter and stammer. Word finding issues become more pronounced. My memory comes and goes.

But I also believe that nothing happens by chance. And I have a faith - at the level of my soul - that all goes as it is supposed to.

Speaking at the conference was a profoundly and unexpectedly spiritual experience. Lots of quiet meditation the night before and a prayer for help, guidance and direction quietly said at the podium. An energy flowed through me that was not my own. Words came unasked for. And an hour passed in a heartbeat, with little recall of what I said. Such is the nature of sharing from the heart. The stories of inspiration from so many others affected by traumatic brain injury left me deeply moved and humbled.

And rather than mourning my loss, Sarah was front and center, her ever-present camera in hand, being a part of our new path together.

Building a "Survivor Family" After Traumatic Brain Injury

"You don't choose your family. They are God's gift to you, as you are to them."
~Desmond Tutu

I'm about to show my age. When I was a kid, I used to love watching TV shows that are now most likely on the TV Oldies Channel. Coming home from school, I'd get out of my school clothes, get into my play clothes and flip on the console sized television. Back in the day, we used to have clothes dedicated school clothes. There I go showing my age again.

A couple of my favorites on afternoon television were *Leave it to Beaver*, and *Father Knows Best*. In the spirit of complete disclosure, though I didn't know it at the time, these were reruns of shows that had aired many years earlier.

Families were pretty traditional back then – both on television and in real life. Dads went to work all day, some moms worked, others stayed home. The family that I grew up in was about as average as you could get. My dad was working in the aerospace industry on the Apollo rocket project while my mom was a middle school math teacher. I grew up with a mom, a dad and 2.0 kids in our family.

Brain injury is a game-changer. It's like having the very foundation of your life torn out – leaving you in the rather unique position of having to rebuild yourself from the ground up. Relationships change and many end completely. Careers change... or end completely. Marriages change... or end tragically. And families can't help but change. It goes with the territory.

During the first couple of years after my own brain injury, if you had asked me my thoughts about how families are impacted by a traumatic brain injury, I would most likely have chimed in that families are fractured and torn apart when a family member sustains a traumatic brain injury.

But as the years pass, I see it for what it really is. Perspectives I have in year five were not possible early on after my brain injury. Looking back with the benefit of hindsight, my family was not fractured. It was slowly being rebuilt as a new kind of family – a *survivor family*.

For the first couple of years, the dust from my cycling accident still filled the air, making any real clarity unattainable. But as the dust settled, and my eyes began to clear, I looked around and realized I was surrounded by a new kind of family. These family members, some knowing and others unaware, have saved my life, have sustained me and have supported me – even during the times I felt like I was unable to support myself.

Long gone is my childhood belief that true family is defined by mother, father, brother and sister who share the same DNA. I have learned to redefine family in the last few years. Looking around with clear eyes, I gaze in true amazement at my new survivor family.

I am one of the fortunate ones as my wife Sarah has been an unwavering member of my family, as have my Mom and Dad. They know and love both David's – the David who was and the David who is. The casualty count has been high as I've lost a few souls very close to me since my accident. But members of this new survivor family continue to do what true family does – love unconditionally.

So, who are these new and unexpected members of my new family? Let's start at the top of my list with fellow TBI survivors. My family first started to grow, with me blissfully unaware, when I started attending a face-to-face support group. We are now in year five of meeting as a support group and many of the members of this group have been part of my life for many, many years. They are family and I love them.

The family circle grows wider with many of those who are now part of my life as a voice for the TBI community. I have come to cherish relationships I have with fellow writers, bloggers, editors and others who at first glance might be perceived to simply be other professionals that I now associate with. But many of these relationships now transcend work. They have become true and steadfast friends. Many of these souls are now part of my new survivor family.

And lest I leave out one of the most unexpected surprises along the way – Facebook. Most anyone who knows me knows that I'm not a shy guy on social media. And I'm glad I'm not. A short ten years ago, there was no way for other survivors to instantly connect with each other. Thankfully those days are gone forever. In fact, I believe that there has never been a better time to be a brain injury survivor. Through a wide range of social outlets, survivors connect instantly – like neurons in a big virtual brain. In a few clicks of a mouse, experiences are validated, new friendships are made and isolation ends.

So many of those who are part of my social circle are now counted as members in good standing of my new survivor family. If I happen to share that it's been a tough day, I am encouraged and supported by others – many of whom I will never meet. Like a traditional family of old, they help support me. And I do what I can to support them. We are all in this together.

These days, having a bit of perspective can be a great thing. No longer am I tempted to look at the glass as half empty. No one recovers from a brain injury on their own. When I take a moment to look at my life – to really see with the eyes of my soul, it's hard not to be grateful for all that I have. I've got one of the largest extended families of anyone I know – an extended family that is my new survivor family.

And if it's worked for me, it can work for you too. There are others, people like me, who are at the ready to be part of your own survivor family.

Metamorphosis

"What the caterpillar calls the end of the world the master calls a butterfly."
~Richard Bach

As a young child, I was always one to shun the mainstream. Not only was this tolerated, it was actually encouraged.

My father has long been one of the best teachers I've had in my life. He did not teach by dictation or rule. No, his was more of an illustrative type of teaching. As a young man, he showed me by living example the importance of living an honorable life.

Daily he would "suit up and show up" for life. Looking back to my life as a child, he would go to work Mondays through Fridays, pay the bills, and do his best to always do the right thing. This was never done for attention, mind you. It was simply the right thing to do, no questions asked.

In the mid 1970's, my dad went through what he has openly called his mid-life crisis. He quit his long-standing job in the aerospace industry, grew out his hair and beard and proceeded to do... well... nothing.

Thankfully, that phase didn't last for long, my mom let him get it out of his system, his employer gratefully took him back on board, and we, as a family, barely missed a heartbeat.

It was during this time that I first noticed a quote hanging on the wall of his bedroom. It was another of those coincidences that leaves me feeling that there is really a Grand Plan in life. The quote was by Henry David Thoreau who has been a literary inspiration to me for the better part of my adult life.

At the age of 12, however, I hadn't a clue about this great visionary.

The quote that hung upon Dad's wall is a concept that should be taught in every school as it is the epitome of tolerance for ones' fellow man.

> *"If a man does not keep pace with his companions, perhaps it is because he hears a different drummer. Let him step to the music which he hears, however measured or far away." ~ Henry David Thoreau*

Here were the words that defined, at least in part, the reality of life as I knew it. Individualism was not only accepted, it was a requisite. Uniqueness was not uncommon. Rather, it was the norm in what amounted to the ultimate oxymoron.

And we come full circle to butterflies and metamorphosis.

For many years, while my pre-adolescent peers were out catching baseballs, I spent my time catching butterflies. No folly here. I had a legitimate child-like wonderment of these amazing and graceful creatures.

In fields and meadows from New Hampshire to Maine and back to Massachusetts, I quietly stalked my prey. My ever-present net in hand, nimble as only a child can be, I patiently waited for the next new discovery to flutter by.

I had butterfly books, butterfly cases, and watched any television show that even remotely had to do with these graceful flyers. When a new catch would come my way, I would preserve them in the types of cases that the entomologists use. You've no doubt seen them in museums with glass in front and cotton batten pressing the butterflies into the glass. My childhood specimens were preserved to this degree of scientific accuracy.

Even today, on the wall of my office hangs one of those cases from my childhood. A Luna moth forever frozen in eternity next to a Tiger Swallowtail; a Viceroy butterfly the constant and silent companion to a Polyphemus moth.

They have survived the passage of time. Mounted perhaps 40 or more years ago, they are a vivid testimonial to my early mounting skills.

It's worth noting that today such an activity would not mesh with my world. I deem all life to be sacred. Other than an errant wasp, most any bug that is lucky enough to get into our home is not squashed. No, they are gently caught and released back into the Wild.

Such was the bliss of youth however, as I had no real awareness that the vital life force that flows through all of us also flowed through my colorful captives.

The entire process of metamorphosis captivated me. Here were caterpillars that had no real beauty, it seemed. They had no awareness of their future and lived in blissful ignorance of what was to become of them.

Chomping on leaves and growing day-by-day, earth-bound by circumstance and not choice, the freedom of flight would be beyond their comprehension.

Yet fly they would. Gracefully. Beautifully. As completely transformed beings.

So it has become with my brain injury. My pre-injury life was akin to the life of the caterpillar. Moving day-by-day, earthbound and living a familiar routine, I had no idea, no comprehension, no way of knowing how much I would change. The veil that blocks our ability to see beyond the moment blocked any inkling of what the future would hold.

Like the caterpillar heading into his cocoon for a long period of darkness and change, so were the months after my accident. My world got immensely small and dark. The light of day was almost entirely blotted out but, within the confines of my own cocoon, I was changing. Like the butterfly, I would be the last to know.

I emerged from my darkness forever changed and vastly different than the being I was before my accident.

Many years ago I read a story that I thought was about a butterfly. As I grow in life experience, I now see that it's really not about a butterfly at all. Rather, it is about the purely human requirement for adversity in life and the ability of life's hardships to not only strengthen us, but to define who we are.

~Book Excerpt, *Metamorphosis, Surviving Brain Injury*.

Post Traumatic Growth

"Grateful people may recover faster from trauma."
~Deborah Norville

Time continues to pass as it inevitably does. Learning about traumatic brain injury has become singularly one of the most fascinating adventures of the newest chapter of my life. The learning process can largely be divided into two parts. First, I continue to learn about daily life as a brain injury survivor every day that I open my eyes. And second, unique opportunities to advocate for those who can't continue to unfold, so often in ways unexpected.

There is no end game in brain injury recovery. Every day, new life situations unfold that I must walk through as a survivor. Tasks and life-events that came with relative ease and fluidity in my life before the injury so often are much more daunting. Daily I suit up and show up for the business of life.

In late 2014, I attended a neurological medical conference in Maine. The conference keynote speaker was a nationally recognized physician and traumatic brain injury book author. Over a decade ago, her own son sustained a brain injury in a tragic hit and run accident. This life-changing event left him with a TBI. His girlfriend was killed by the same hit-and-run driver.

Like so many others that I now call friends, the conference speaker learned about traumatic brain injury by circumstance, being thrown into this new and so often unpredictable life by fate. It was during her keynote presentation that a stunning revelation was made. In attendance at the conference were members of the medical and professional community. Attendees also included many brain injury survivors.

From the podium, the bombshell was dropped. "We, as members of the medical community, got it wrong when we told you the most recovery would happen within the first two years after a brain injury," she stated with firm and unquestionable conviction. "Members of the medical community used the two year number because that is about how long we monitored most survivors."

The crowd of attendees sat there in stunned silence. To many within the professional community, this may have come as new news. But to those who live daily with a brain injury, we had just had our own experiences validated. Over the years since my own injury, I have heard so many others share that gains, measurable gains, have been made many years after the original injury.

This is not as new a revelation as some think. In her 2009 title, *My Stroke of Insight*, Dr. Jill Bolte-Taylor speaks of what she calls "measurable gains," occurring up to nine years after her injury. And while the timeline of recovery is as unique as the individual, an increasing number of medical professionals are now rewriting the book on the brain injury recovery timeline. This should come as exciting news to those who have been told otherwise.

It's during times like these that the first year diagnosis of "permanent disability" come back to haunt me. Though a trusted and respected neuropsychologist, his thinking was still of the old-school persuasion. Just as every brain injury is different, so can be the wide range of understanding within the medical community.

So much of my life has been spent in learning how to live what amounts to a second life. From books to websites, from science channel specials to smart phone apps, there is a veritable wellspring of information about brain injury available. And while I've quickly learned that you can't believe everything you see or read, there is no shortage of meaningful information.

Somewhere during my second year as a survivor, I was introduced to a concept that was entirely new to me. In fact, it was such an alien concept, that it almost didn't make sense. For the first time ever, I heard the term "Post Traumatic Growth."

"Post Traumatic Growth refers to positive psychological change experienced as a result of the struggle with highly challenging life circumstances. These sets of circumstances represent significant challenges to the adaptive resources of the individual, and pose significant challenges to individuals' way of understanding the world and their place in it.

Post Traumatic Growth is not about returning to the same life as it was previously experienced before a period of traumatic suffering; but rather it is about undergoing significant 'life-changing' psychological shifts in thinking and relating to the world, that contribute to a personal process of change, that is deeply meaningful." (Source: Wikipedia.org)

Reading through this as well as other resources about Post Traumatic Growth, it became increasingly clear that there were changes coming to pass in my own life that were on the positive side of the ledger. While it can be all too easy to focus on how much my brain injury has cost me and those close to me, it was time to begin shifting my focus. I began to look more closely at the positive that was coming to pass since my accident.

This was clearly a tall-order task. For several years, I viewed my injury as a "taker." It took away my sense of self, it removed many of my closest friendships, our financial security melted like an early spring snow. It was the gift that kept on taking.

Through it all, my wife Sarah shared her own personal mantra over and over. "The curse will become a blessing." While I believed that might come to pass in her life, how could it possibly come to pass in my own? After all, I was the one with the injury!

Brain injury is indeed a game-changer. For so many living with a brain injury, the world gets smaller. Family dynamics change and life as we knew it is gone.

Brain injury and isolation go hand-in-hand. Personality changes, dwindling finances, and a host of other complications can lead to an almost shut-in existence for many survivors. Brain injury is a family affair that, in reality, directly impacts anyone close to the survivor.

As recently as a decade ago, there was no real way for survivors, or those who love them, to connect with each other easily and conveniently. Sure, face-to-face support groups have been around for a very long time. They remain a veritable lifeline for survivors and family members to connect.

But most face-to-face support group meetings are held on a monthly basis. Support group meetings are like an oasis in the midst of a desert, but survivors were relegated to long periods of time with minimal direct contact with each other. I know this from firsthand experience. Prior to my own traumatic brain injury, I didn't even have a nodding acquaintance with it. I never knowingly met one of the several million people who live daily with a brain injury. Any news accounts about the prevalence of brain injury in today's world fell on deaf ears. Somehow I had missed the proverbial memo about that.

I found myself completely and utterly alone after my own injury. For months, I muddled through my day-to-day existence never knowing that there were so many others who shared my fate, others who unknowingly held the key to the end of my isolation.

There is a healing, camaraderie, an indescribable bond that happens among survivors.

At my face-to-face support group, I heard others share about the same daily struggles I was living with. Better still, as the years passed and we grew stronger as a group, compensatory strategies were shared and that sense of isolation evaporated—at least for an hour or so a month.

However, in my own life, there was still a void. Weeks without regular contact with other survivors took its toll. In my life before brain injury, much of my work professionally was Internet-based. So it came as a surprise to no one that it was to the Internet that I turned again.

No one was more surprised than me to find a vibrant and thriving web-based community of people affected by brain injury. From online survivor groups to Facebook groups of all kinds, here were people from around the globe who were communicating with each other on a daily basis.

Gone was the blackout window of weeks between connecting with others who shared my fate. While not quite as intimate as my monthly support group meetings, I was able to connect with so many others with the simple click of a mouse.

I am blessed that my internal compass still points in the positive direction. When living with a brain injury, attitude really is everything. Knowing that a positive outlook can really make life easier as a survivor, I made the decision to jump into the ring. In 2013, I founded what I had envisioned to be a smaller online community, TBI Hope & Inspiration.

My intent was to offer what amounted to a daily positive thought or story about how to live after a brain injury. I underestimated two things: the power of the Internet and the soul-level need for other survivors to connect with each other. Within a year, this "small" group blossomed to over 10,000 members from around the world.

Like people, online groups have very unique personalities. Weekly, members ask me to post questions to the group and the response is overwhelming. When a member posts a question about most any aspect of life after brain injury, others chime in to share their own experiences — often within minutes.

And here is where the real miracle begins to take form. So many people living with a TBI have mobility challenges. Many do not drive and many have shared over the years that they don't have access to a local support group. Yet these same people are willing to share their lives as survivors so that others can be helped.

Each member who contributes does so with the intent to help but comes away from the experience feeling better knowing that they have positively impacted someone's life. Their own heavy load is lightened, and they see that their experience as survivors makes them uniquely useful to help others. Their lives are enriched by the very act of giving.

This same spirit can be found in other online groups as well as websites the world over. Living my life as a brain injury survivor remains the toughest challenge of my existence. But when I take a moment to step back and look at how fortunate I am to be able to instantly connect with others, it's difficult not to be grateful.

My own experience as one who lives a life impacted became the catalyst to help thousands of others with similar lives the world over. Over the years, many group members have expressed gratitude for finding this Facebook community. Many have shared that the posts, the short stories and the comments from other members have let them know that they were not alone - that there were others who shared similar circumstances.

Where I had initially come to these communities as a "taker," reading with little or no comment, as time passed, I began to give back to those who had so freely offered to help others. From a thriving Facebook community to regular blogging, from numerous articles that saw international distribution, I had found my new voice and wasn't afraid to use it.

Had I not been injured, so many of these same people would not have found the end of the isolation they knew. My own "curse" became their "blessing." Though it doesn't always take away the many challenges at hand, simply knowing that others are helped by my sharing does so much to lighten the load. Weekly, other survivors from around the world reach out to me to express thanks. I find it humbling and unexpected. Comments like this drive me to continue my advocacy work. Past history has shown clearly that others are helped. Perhaps even you.

In 2013, a neurological medical convention conference committee reached out to me. One of the committee members knew of my story and how far I had progressed. I was invited to present as the keynote speaker. In sharing the news with my dad, I let him know that I normally play connect-the-dots with life experiences, but that I had no point of reference for my upcoming speaking engagement.

"David, this is the first dot," he shared with his sage wisdom. My dad has always said so much with so few words. There are some who no doubt think I could learn a bit from him.

Knees quaking, hands sweating and voice trembling I took to the podium... and have never looked back. Looking down, in real time, as real people who were either impacted by brain injury, or were there to support those of us who have been, was an experience I will forever cherish. I was scheduled to speak for an hour. An hour and ten minutes later, my presentation ended with applause that overwhelmed me. Over the course of the afternoon that followed, so many people thanked me for putting a face, and a voice, on the human side of brain injury. We are survivors, not statistics.

Since that first presentation, I have had the opportunity to share with numerous survivors throughout New England. And my goals are always the same: be painfully open, brutally honest and sincere. This I do out of a deep, soul-level feeling that I owe it to those who take time out of their day to listen. Survivors come away feeling less alone, and members of the medical and professional community have openly shared that they have a new and deeper understanding of what we, as survivors face.

Time after time over the last few years, I have been overwhelmed with the feeling that my life is supposed to unfold as it has, and that my experience as a true survivor has offered a God-given opportunity to serve others so that the greater good is realized. To think that I had given serious thought to suicide during that abysmally tough first year and have moved on to a place where this very unique life experience can be used as a mechanism to help others is remarkable.

Many years ago, I heard someone say that nothing happens by mistake. I was a younger man and a skeptic. Someone loses a child, or a parent to a senseless accident? How can this be part of a grander plan? A young child passes from losing a battle with cancer and you want me to believe that life happens the way it's supposed to? One of my closest friends lost a son many years ago. He is now drawn toward and comforts those with similar losses. Fate has put many others in his path who have lost children. He shares from his own personal experience and others come away with lighter loads because of it.

In this light, is it really that much of a leap to believe that my life was spared that fated day so that I could, at least in part, help others? Yes, I believe this from within the depths of my soul. If you have a heartbeat, you have experienced some type of human tragedy. This I know as surely as I know that the sun will rise and set over today. I encourage you to share your story with others walking the same path. From your own personal tragedy will come triumph. If it happened to me, it can happen to you.

Afterword

Many years ago I heard words that made me cringe.

"Recovery from a brain injury is lifelong."

No longer does this bother me. I've learned that time is now my friend. I have new adventures awaiting and new lessons to learn.

If you've found my experiences to be helpful as you walk your own life's path, I encourage you to please offer a book review on Amazon.com.

As my own life as a survivor continues to unfold, I will continue to live transparently as I chronicle life as a brain injury survivor. Be sure for follow my blog at www.DavidsNewLife.com

Peace to you as your own journey continues.

~D

www.ingramcontent.com/pod-product-compliance
Lightning Source LLC
Chambersburg PA
CBHW051908170526
45168CB00001B/288